Team Leadership and Partnering in Nursing and Health Care

Cynthia Armstrong Persily, PhD, RN, FAAN, holds the dual position of associate dean, Graduate Practice Programs, and chairperson–Charleston Division at the West Virginia University School of Nursing. Since 2006, Dr. Persily has served as executive director of the West Virginia Nursing Leadership Institute, a program to develop teams of nurses to provide leadership in a changing health care environment. Dr. Persily serves as the deputy director of the West Virginia Rural Health Research Center, where she has focused on workforce research, recently completing a study on delineating the current health care workforce supply in West Virginia. She is a Fellow of the American Academy of Nursing. Dr. Persily was named a Robert Wood Johnson Executive Nurse Fellow in 2001 and recently concluded a 3-year term as an appointed member of the National Advisory Council for that program. Dr. Persily is active in professional leadership, previously serving as founding chairperson of the West Virginia Center for Nursing, and currently as the chairperson of the center's research and data committee, which collects, analyzes, and disseminates data relative to the nursing workforce. As a previous member, secretary, and president of the West Virginia Board of Examiners for Registered Professional Nurses, Dr. Persily provided leadership for nursing regulation. Lastly, she serves in leadership roles on a number of community boards.

Team Leadership and Partnering in Nursing and Health Care

Cynthia Armstrong Persily, PhD, RN, FAAN

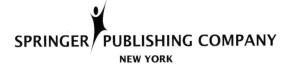

SPRINGER PUBLISHING COMPANY
NEW YORK

Springer Publishing Company, LLC
11 West 42nd Street
New York, NY 10036
www.springerpub.com

Acquisitions Editor: Margaret Zuccarini
Composition: Techset

ISBN: 978-0-8261-9988-1
e-book ISBN: 978-0-8261-9989-8

13 14 15 16 / 5 4 3 2 1

The author and the publisher of this Work have made every effort to use sources believed to be reliable to provide information that is accurate and compatible with the standards generally accepted at the time of publication. Because medical science is continually advancing, our knowledge base continues to expand. Therefore, as new information becomes available, changes in procedures become necessary. We recommend that the reader always consult current research and specific institutional policies before performing any clinical procedure. The author and publisher shall not be liable for any special, consequential, or exemplary damages resulting, in whole or in part, from the readers' use of, or reliance on, the information contained in this book. The publisher has no responsibility for the persistence or accuracy of URLs for external or third-party Internet websites referred to in this publication and does not guarantee that any content on such websites is, or will remain, accurate or appropriate.

Library of Congress Cataloging-in-Publication Data

Persily, Cynthia Armstrong.
 Team leadership and partnering in nursing and health care / Cynthia Armstrong Persily.
     p. ; cm.
 Includes bibliographical references and index.
 ISBN 978-0-8261-9988-1 — ISBN 978-0-8261-9989-8 (e-book)
 I. Title.
 [DNLM: 1. Leadership. 2. Nursing—organization & administration.
3. Delivery of Health Care—organization & administration.
4. Interprofessional Relations. WY 105]
 RT89.3
 362.17'3068--dc23

                                                                                    2013006888

Printed in the United States of America by Bang Printing.

Contents

Section III Nursing and Health Care Team Issues and Challenges

Section IV Leverage of Nursing and Health Care Team Results

Preface

*T*he work of teams is essential in ensuring positive health outcomes. However, the skills necessary to lead and work as a team
are not innate—but rather are all too often learned through trial and
error. In 2006, I was privileged to establish the West Virginia Nursing
Leadership Institute (WVNLI), designed to provide nurses with the
leadership skills they need for the future. After 3 years of training
individual nurses, the staff of WVNLI made an important observation. Those organizations that supported groups of nurses attending
the year-long training program, whose nurses then went back to their
organizations armed with leadership knowledge, skills, and competencies, were much more likely to be transformed by the leadership
of that group of nurses than organizations that only supported one
nurse attending the program. Those individual nurses went back to
their organizations armed with the same knowledge, skills, and competencies, but were much less likely to be able to lead change in the
organization. Why? One consultant called it the "clean fish in a dirty
pond" syndrome—the nurse had changed, but the organization had
not, and that nurse did not have a peer group with similar knowledge,
skills, and attitudes to join forces for change. We decided to use that
revelation to transform the program into a team development program—bringing teams of nurses from various organizations to learn,
to develop as a team, and to use their new skills in team leadership to
influence the direction of their organization and to mentor other teams
in their development. This book is based on what we all learned on
that journey—how to prepare teams to effectively lead transformation
in their organizations, communities, and beyond.

—*Cynthia Armstrong Persily, PhD, RN, FAAN*

Acknowledgments

*B*ecause the work that was accomplished at the West Virginia Nursing Leadership Institute (WVNLI) was integral to the development of this text, I must acknowledge the support and effort of a number of individuals and groups who allowed the WVNLI initiative to be successful. First, I acknowledge West Virginia University, which has offered me immeasurable support in my scholarly endeavors. Without the gift of time, the dream of this book would not have become a reality. I must recognize a number of philanthropic organizations that supported the work of WVNLI because without their support we could not have survived: the Claude Worthington Benedum Foundation, the Northwest Health Foundation/Robert Wood Johnson Foundation Partners Investing in Nursing's Future program and, most important, our local partner, the Greater Kanawha Valley Foundation, which helped us to garner additional support. These organizations did not just give us funds, but rather, they joined our team, and for that I will be forever grateful. Next, I would like to acknowledge the support of the advisory board for WVNLI, made up of leaders in health care and business from across our state. Their ideas, encouragement, and support allow the institute to flourish. I would be remiss if I did not also recognize the immense support offered by local health care institutions to the institute through their support of the nurse participants. The visionary organizational leaders of these institutions realize the importance of team leadership training and the potential that this training holds for their organization, and invest even when health care dollars are in short supply. And finally, I must highlight the nurses who participated so fully in the WVNLI experience. Your experiences as you completely engaged and immersed yourselves in learning about teams, teamwork, and leadership culminated in the development of this book. Sharing your challenges and your successes inspires me—and I hope this book captures a bit of what we have all learned together on that journey.

Nursing and Health Care Team Models and Skills

The Intersection of Teams, Partnerships, and Leadership in Nursing and Health Care

Talent wins games, but teamwork and intelligence win championships.
—Michael Jordan

LEARNING OBJECTIVES

1. Define "team" in the context of nursing and health care.
2. Discuss the importance of partnerships in modern health care.
3. Analyze the impact of teams and partnerships in health care today.
4. Identify how nursing education at a variety of levels prepares nurses with teamwork competencies.
5. Illustrate the importance of team competencies to interprofessional practice.

*H*ow many of us have been a member of a team? Think back over the course of your life and your professional career, and you will likely identify multiple team memberships—teams for school projects, sports teams, care teams, special project teams, and administrative or leadership teams will probably be a part of your list. How many of us have been members of a partnership? Again, think about your personal and professional life. Perhaps your list will include a significant relationship, a marriage, a partnership across departments, or across organizations. But what do all of these teams and partnerships have in common? This book will provide you with an understanding of the common features of teams and partnerships, and is designed to help you develop the competencies needed to intentionally create and lead effective teams and partnerships. The book is based on the belief that skills in teaming and partnering are translatable to any health care situation, and if these skills are mastered, more effective teams and partnerships, regardless of their purpose, will result. Throughout the book, you will find case examples from a variety of nursing and health care situations that will illustrate the competencies. These case studies are drawn from direct care environments such as hospitals, long-term care and public health, education settings, management and administrative environments, and even public policy. Through these case studies, you will see competencies in action, providing you with a context for application of team and partnering skills in your environment.

WHAT IS A TEAM IN NURSING AND HEALTH CARE?

Although the nursing and health care literature is replete with praise for teamwork, many experts have faulted research in the area of teamwork because of a lack of a common definition of the concepts of *team* and *teamwork*. A simple definition of *team* found in the *Merriam-Webster Dictionary* (2011) is "a number of persons associated together in work or activity." Katzenbach and Smith (1993) have posited that a team is "a small number of people with complementary skills, committed to a common purpose, performance goals, and approach for which they hold themselves mutually accountable" (p. 45). Mickan (2005) agrees, calling a team "a small manageable number of members with the appropriate mix of expertise, who are committed to a meaningful purpose for which they are collectively responsible" (p. 211). Using these definitions, teams could be characterized as having some common traits:

- Small group of members
- Complementary skills, mixed expertise
- Agreed-upon purpose for existence as a team
- Collective accountability and responsibility

Teamwork, or the work of teams, is seen in modern health care as an important facilitator of positive outcomes. How does teamwork relate to the commonly defined traits of teams? The *Merriam-Webster Dictionary* (2011) defines *teamwork* as "work done by several associates with each doing a part but all subordinating personal prominence to the efficiency of the whole." This definition provides some insight into the actions that may lead to collective accountability and responsibility, specifically the importance of the success of the team over the importance of any one individual team member's status. But what else is necessary for a team to be successful in its work? After an analysis of the concept of teamwork in health care, Xyrichis and Ream (2008) proposed that teamwork be defined as a "dynamic process involving two or more health care professionals with complementary backgrounds and skills, sharing common health goals and exercising concerted physical and mental effort in assessing, planning or evaluating patient care. This is accomplished through interdependent collaboration, open communication and shared decision-making, and generates value-added patient, organizational, and staff outcomes" (p. 238). This definition provides us with insights into the necessary actions of a team in order to affect positive outcomes. So, we could add the following actions involved in a team's work to our list of common team traits:

- Interdependence
- Collaboration
- Open and frank communication
- Shared decision making

WHAT IS A PARTNERSHIP IN NURSING AND HEALTH CARE?

A term closely related to *team* and *teamwork* is *partnership*. The Institute of Medicine (IOM), in the 2010 report *The Future of Nursing: Leading Change, Advancing Health*, has called for new partnerships to ensure that we have enough nurses and nurses with the right skills and competencies to care for society in the future (pp. 250–251). The *Oxford Dictionary* (2011) defines *partnership* within the context of acting as a partner, which is defined as "a person who takes part in an undertaking with another or others, especially in a business or firm with shared risks and profits." Similar then to teaming, partnerships imply shared responsibilities and accountability. Perhaps a more fitting definition of partnerships for health care is one proposed by the World Health Organization, which defines a partnership as "a collaborative relationship between two or more parties based on trust, equality and mutual understanding for the achievement of a specified goal. Partnerships involve risks as well as benefits, making shared accountability critical" (WHO, 2009, p. 2). Many times partnerships are considered to be interorganizational, as opposed to teams, which are typically considered to be intraorganizational. However, these rules do not always hold, and teams and partnerships are more likely defined by their common characteristics and context as opposed to their locations and members.

Just as teams have common characteristics and traits, so do partnerships. Successful partnerships require specific skills and strategies. The common traits found in the definitions of partnership presented here include:

- Collaboration
- Trust
- Equality
- Mutual understanding
- A stated goal
- Shared accountability

Although there are many additional definitions of teams, teamwork, and partnership in the literature, the definitions presented in this chapter provide us with the common traits of teams and partnerships that will serve as a framework for discussions later in this book about building teams, strategies for team success, working as a team within organizations, facilitating change, the evaluation of team outcomes, and finally, special considerations for building partnerships in health care.

HOW DO TEAMS AND PARTNERSHIPS IMPACT 21ST-CENTURY HEALTH CARE?

Now that we have a shared understanding of teams and partnerships, the question remains, why are teams and partnerships so important in 21st-century health care? Multiple reports, articles, and books have been written about the impact of teams and partnerships in health care over the last two decades. Teams in health care have been credited with positive impacts on the safety and quality of care, job satisfaction and decreased burnout and turnover, and organizational success.

Safety and Quality of Care

Organizations such as the IOM (1999), the Agency for HealthCare Quality and Research (AHRQ), The Joint Commission, and the Centers for Medicaid and Medicare Services (CMS) have advocated for the use of teams in health care as a method to improve patient safety and quality of care. In relation to patient safety, fewer errors occur when teamwork is strong because processes are planned and standardized. Members know their responsibilities as well as the responsibilities of their teammates. Team members are aware of the actions of their teammates, and notice errors before they occur. Effective team members trust others' judgment, have mutual respect, and pay attention to one another's safety concerns (IOM, 1999). A Cochrane systematic review of the benefits of teamwork in 2007 found that practice-based interprofessional team interventions improve health care delivery and outcomes, but the small number of studies, small sample size, and challenges in measuring collaboration make it difficult to generalize about the elements of teamwork that were responsible for these positive effects (Zwarenstein, Goldman, & Reeves, 2009). A review of the literature on the benefits of team approaches from 1985 through 2004 found that the diversity of clinical expertise involved in team decision making may account for improvements in patient care and organizational effectiveness, while collaboration, conflict resolution, participation, and cohesion may enhance team member satisfaction and perceptions of team effectiveness (Lemieux-Charles & McGuire, 2006). Specific safety and quality outcomes that have been documented to be impacted by teamwork include mortality rates (Langhorne, Williams, Gilchrist, & Howie, 1993), operative complications and death (Mazzocco et al., 2009), and patient satisfaction (Meterko, Mohr, & Young, 2004). Higher teamwork scores have been associated with higher levels of nurse assessed quality of care, perceived quality improvement over the last year, and confidence that patients could manage their care when discharged (Rafferty, Ball, & Aiken, 2001). Specifically, team care in a wide variety of clinical settings has been associated with the following outcomes: decreased length of hospital stay (Barker et al., 1985); increased functional capacity in older adults, improved mental status, decreased falls, improved self-perceived health and life satisfaction, and reduced hospital readmission rates in community-dwelling elders (Johannson, Eklund, & Gosman-Hedstro, 2010); fewer nursing home admissions following hospitalization (Zimmer, Groth-Junker, & McClusker, 1985); decreased mortality 1 year after discharge (Langhorne et al., 1993); decreased prescribing of psychotropic drugs among nursing home residents in Sweden (Schmidt, Claesson, Westerholm, Nilsson, & Svarstad, 1998); an increase in maternal transfusions attributed to more rapid identification of hemorrhage (Contratti, Ng, & Deeb, 2012); and decreased overall health care costs (Williams, Williams,

Zimmer, Hall, & Podgorski, 1987). A British report revealed that a lack of communication and teamwork within the obstetric and midwifery teams and in multidisciplinary teamwork contributed to substandard care resulting in over half of the maternal deaths they examined in a 2-year period (Lewis & Drife, 2004). A supportive practice environment, which includes many markers of effective teamwork such as effective participation by nurses in hospital affairs teams and collegial nurse–physician relationships, has been documented to positively correlate with nurse's error-interception practices, resulting in fewer medication errors (Flynn, Liang, Dickson, Xie, & Suh, 2012).

Job Turnover, Burnout, and Retention

Nurses have long recognized the satisfaction that comes from working with an effective team. Teams have been documented to promote job satisfaction for team members (Gage, 1998). But teamwork has even greater impact on nurses' lives than mere satisfaction. In a study by Rafferty et al. (2001), nurses in England with higher teamwork scores were not only significantly more likely to be satisfied with their jobs, but they planned to stay in those jobs, and had lower burnout scores. Nurses with higher teamwork scores also exhibited higher levels of autonomy and were more involved in decision making. An intervention to increase teamwork in an acute care hospital by Kalisch, Curley, and Stefanov (2007) resulted in lower staff turnover and vacancy rates. In a study of nurses intent on leaving their current positions, Larrabee and colleagues (2003) found that the major predictor of intent to leave was job dissatisfaction, and the major predictor of job satisfaction was psychological empowerment. Predictors of psychological empowerment identified in this study included, among others, the essential teamwork characteristics of nurse/physician collaboration and group cohesion. As a nursing workforce crisis continues in the United States, nurse leaders are increasingly looking to teams and teamwork to improve nurse job satisfaction and retention.

Organizational Success

Organizational outcomes are increasingly dependent upon teams and teamwork. High-reliability organizations, like those in health care as well as other industries like aviation and the military, rely on finely tuned teams for organizational success. Organizations that are "hypercomplex, tightly coupled (i.e. task interdependence), hierarchical, time compressed, and rely upon synchronized outcomes" (Baker, Day, & Salas, 2006, p. 1590) are especially dependent upon teamwork. It has long been recognized in other industries that teamwork, and in fact the tenure of the team relationship, has an impact on organizational outcomes such as strategy and performance, which exceeds industry performance (Finkelstein & Hambrick, 1990). Other researchers have shown that top management teams have significant impact on other organizational outcomes, such as strategic change (Cho & Hambrick, 2006; Wiersema & Bantel, 1992) and innovation (Bantel & Jackson, 1989; Elenkov, Judge, & Wright, 2005; Smith & Tushman, 2005). However, it is increasingly evident that teams across the organization are as important as management teams to organizational success. In a multi-industry survey conducted by the Center for Creative Leadership, 91% of respondents identified teams as a key ingredient to organizational success (Center for Creative Leadership, 2007). Collaborative nurse practitioner and physician hospitalist teams have been documented to decrease length of stay and costs and increase hospital profits with readmission and mortality rates similar to traditional care models (Cowan et al., 2006; Ettner et al., 2006). Partnerships linking teams of nurses and finance department members in one university hospital significantly improved organizational outcomes, including managing growth and budget variances, and improving interpreter services for the organization (Esposito-Herr, Persinger, Regier, & Hunt, 2009).

HOW WILL NURSES AND OTHER HEALTH CARE PROVIDERS LEARN TO WORK IN 21ST-CENTURY TEAMS?

Organizations such as the IOM have called for teamwork training. Accrediting bodies like the Joint Commission on Accreditation of Healthcare Organizations (JCAHO, now referred to as The Joint Commission) and others require teamwork competencies to realize patient care quality and safety goals. Just as multiple organizations have advocated for the use of teams to improve care processes, academic organizations have begun to recognize the need for the integration of teamwork competencies into entry-level and continuing-education efforts. Teamwork competencies and education standards are now commonplace for education-accrediting bodies.

In nursing education, teamwork competencies are now included across all levels of nursing education accreditation standards. The

National League for Nursing (NLN) includes teamwork as an integrating concept for nursing curricula for graduates of nursing programs at all levels, from practical nursing through the doctorate (NLN, 2010) (Figure 1.1).

The American Association of Colleges of Nursing (AACN), in their *The Essentials for Master's Education in Nursing* series, outline the necessary curriculum content and expected competencies of graduates from baccalaureate, master's, and Doctor of Nursing Practice programs. At each level of education, teamwork is specifically noted as an essential curricular component. For instance, at the baccalaureate level, "leadership skills are needed that emphasize ethical and critical decision making, initiating and maintaining effective working relationships, using mutually respectful communication and collaboration within inter-professional teams, care coordination, delegation, and developing conflict resolution strategies" are key competencies for graduates (Essentials of Baccalaureate Education, 2008, p. 13). Specific to teamwork, the AACN believes that baccalaureate graduates are prepared to "apply leadership concepts, skills, and decision making in the provision of high quality nursing care, health care team coordination, and the oversight and accountability

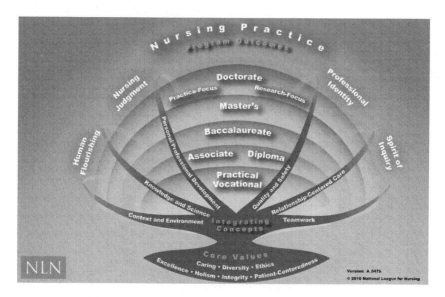

FIGURE 1.1 NLN education competencies model.
Source: Reprinted with permission of National League for Nursing (2010).

for care delivery in a variety of settings" and to "demonstrate leadership and communication skills to effectively implement patient safety and quality improvement initiatives within the context of the inter-professional team" (p. 14). Education experiences should develop these competencies in baccalaureate graduates and might include content and clinical experiences to build "teamwork skills, including effective teams/characteristics, application to patient care teams, team process, conflict resolution, delegation, supervision, and collaboration" (p. 15). The AACN advocates for building knowledge regarding teamwork at the graduate level of nursing education. *The Essentials for Master's Education in Nursing* (2011) holds that master's graduates must be "able to demonstrate leadership by initiating and maintaining effective working relationships using mutually respectful communication and collaboration within inter-professional teams, demonstrating skills in care coordination, delegation, and initiating conflict resolution strategies" (p. 11). Again, specific to teamwork, the AACN believes that MSN degree programs should prepare graduates who are qualified to "apply leadership skills and decision making in the provision of culturally responsive, high-quality nursing care, health care team coordination, and the oversight and accountability for care delivery and outcomes" and "assume a leadership role in effectively implementing patient safety and quality improvement initiatives within the context of the interprofessional team using effective communication (scholarly writing, speaking, and group interaction) skills" (p. 12). Education experiences should prepare graduates with these competencies, and may include content regarding "teams and teamwork, including team leadership, building effective teams, and nurturing teams" (p. 13). Finally, at the clinical doctorate level, the AACN Essentials of Doctoral Education for Advanced Practice Nursing (2006) holds that the Doctor of Nursing Practice (DNP) graduate has "advanced preparation in the inter-professional dimension of health care that enables them to facilitate collaborative team functioning and overcome impediments to inter-professional practice … and DNP graduates have preparation in methods of effective team leadership and are prepared to play a central role in establishing inter-professional teams, participating in the work of the team, and assuming leadership of the team when appropriate" (p. 14). Education programs should prepare DNP graduates to "lead inter-professional teams in the analysis of complex practice and organizational issues" and "employ consultative and leadership skills with intra-professional and inter-professional teams to create change in health care and complex health care delivery systems" (p. 15).

The Quality and Safety Education for Nurses (QSEN) initiative, funded by the Robert Wood Johnson Foundation, is a national initiative to transform nursing education to integrate quality and safety competencies. QSEN clearly emphasizes the need for teamwork and collaboration as a quality and safety imperative for nursing education at the pre-licensure and advanced nursing practice levels. Integral knowledge, skills, and attitudes for teamwork and collaboration have been developed, and are now being adopted into a variety of nursing programs (QSEN, 2012). The KSAs (knowledge, skills, and attitudes) for pre-licensure programs are shown in Table 1.1, and for Advanced Nursing Practice in Table 1.2. For more information on the QSEN initiative, including competencies, teaching strategies, and additional resources, please visit their website at www.qsen.org.

Most recently, in May of 2011, the Interprofessional Education Collaboration (IPEC) released a report of an expert panel, convened to determine core competencies for interprofessional collaborative practice (Interprofessional Education Collaborative Expert Panel, 2011). The IPEC is sponsored by associations that lead health professions education in the United States, including the American Association of Colleges of Nursing, the American Association of Colleges of Osteopathic Medicine, the American Association of Colleges of Pharmacy, the American Dental Education Association, the Association of American Medical Colleges, and the Association of Schools of Public Health. The Expert Panel's report titled "Core Competencies for Interprofessional Collaborative Practice" (2011) concluded that there were four essential domains of competencies for interprofessional practice. These include Competency Domain 1: Values/Ethics for Interprofessional Practice; Competency Domain 2: Roles/Responsibilities; Competency Domain 3: Interprofessional Communication; and Competency Domain 4: Teams and Teamwork. Through a consensus process, the expert panel determined 11 essential competencies to support effective teams. The general competency statement for the domain of teams and teamwork is that all health care providers should be able to "apply relationship-building values and the principles of team dynamics to perform effectively in different team roles to plan and deliver patient-/population-centered care that is safe, timely, efficient, effective, and equitable" (IPEC, 2011,

TABLE 1.1
Teamwork and Collaboration Knowledge, Skills, and Attitudes for Pre-Licensure Education

KNOWLEDGE	SKILLS	ATTITUDES
Describe own strengths, limitations, and values in functioning as a member of a team	Demonstrate awareness of own strengths and limitations as a team member Initiate plan for self-development as a team member Act with integrity, consistency, and respect for differing views	
Describe scopes of practice and roles of all health care team members	Function competently within own scope of practice as a member of the health care team	Value the perspectives and expertise of all health team members
Describe strategies for identifying and managing overlaps in team member roles and accountabilities	Assume role of team member or leader based on the situation Initiate requests for help when appropriate to situation	Respect the centrality of the patient/family as core members of any health care team
Recognize contributions of other individuals and groups in helping patient/family achieve health goals	Clarify roles and accountabilities under conditions of potential overlap in team member functioning Integrate the contributions of others who play a role in helping patients and families achieve health goals	Respect the unique attributes that members bring to a team, including variations in professional orientations and accountabilities
Analyze differences in communication style preferences among patients and families, nurses, and other members of the health care team	Communicate with team members, adapting own style of communicating to needs of the team and situation Demonstrate commitment to team goals	Value teamwork and the relationships upon which it is based

(continued)

TABLE 1.1
Teamwork and Collaboration Knowledge, Skills, and
Attitudes for Pre-Licensure Education (*continued*)

KNOWLEDGE	SKILLS	ATTITUDES
Describe impact of own communication style on others Discuss effective strategies for communicating and resolving conflict	Solicit input from other team members to improve individual, as well as team, performance	Value different styles of communication used by patients, families, and health care providers
	Initiate actions to resolve conflict	Contribute to resolution of conflict and disagreement
Describe examples of the impact of team functioning on safety and quality of care	Follow communication practices that minimize risks associated with handoffs among providers and across transitions of care	Appreciate the risks associated with handoffs among providers and across transitions of care
Explain authority gradients and their influence on teamwork and patient safety	Follow communication styles that diminish the risks associated with authority gradients among team members Assert own position/ perspective and supporting evidence in discussions about patient care	
Identify system barriers and facilitators of effective team functioning	Participate in designing systems that support effective teamwork	Value the influence of system solutions in achieving team functioning
Examine strategies for improving systems to support team functioning		

Note: Definition of teamwork and collaboration competency: Function effectively within nursing and interprofessional teams, fostering open communication, mutual respect, and shared decision making to achieve quality patient care.

Source: Reprinted from Cronenwett et al. (2007), with permission from Elsevier.

TABLE 1.2
Teamwork and Collaboration Knowledge, Skills, and
Attitudes for Advanced Practice Nursing Education

KNOWLEDGE	SKILLS	ATTITUDES
Analyze own strengths, limitations, and values as a member of the team Analyze impact of own advanced practice role and its contributions to team functioning	Demonstrate awareness of own strengths and limitations as a team member Continuously plan for improvement in use of self in effective team development and functioning	Acknowledge own contributions to effective or ineffective team functioning
Describe scopes of practice and roles of all health care team members	Act with integrity, consistency, and respect for differing views Function competently within own scope of practice as a member of the health care team	Respect the unique attributes that members bring to a team, including variation in professional orientations, competencies, and accountabilities
Analyze strategies for identifying and managing overlaps in team member roles and accountabilities	Assume role of team member or leader based on the situation Guide the team in managing areas of overlap in team member functioning Solicit input from other team members to improve individual, as well as team, performance Empower contributions of others who play a role in helping patients and families achieve health goals	Respect the centrality of the patient/family as core members of any health care team
Analyze strategies that influence the ability to initiate and sustain effective partnerships with members of nursing and inter-professional teams	Initiate and sustain effective health care teams	Appreciate importance of interprofessional collaboration

(continued)

TABLE 1.2
Teamwork and Collaboration Knowledge, Skills, and Attitudes
for Advanced Practice Nursing Education (*continued*)

KNOWLEDGE	SKILLS	ATTITUDES
Analyze impact of cultural diversity on team functioning	Communicate with team members, adapting own style of communicating to needs of the team and situation	Value collaboration with nurses and other members of the nursing team
Analyze differences in communication style preferences among patients and families, advanced practice nurses, and other members of the health care team	Communicate respect for team member competence in communication	Value different styles of communication
Describe impact of own communication style on others	Initiate actions to resolve conflict	
Describe examples of the impact of team functioning on safety and quality of care	Follow communication practices that minimize risks associated with handoffs among providers and across transitions of care	Appreciate the risks associated with handoffs among providers and across transitions of care
Analyze authority gradients and their influence on teamwork and patient safety	Choose communication styles that diminish the risks associated with authority gradients among team members	Value the solutions obtained through systematic, inter-professional collaborative efforts
	Assert own position/ perspective and supporting evidence in discussions about patient care	
Identify system barriers and facilitators of effective team functioning	Lead or participate in the design and implementation of systems that support effective teamwork	Value the influence of system solutions in achieving team functioning

(*continued*)

TABLE 1.2
Teamwork and Collaboration Knowledge, Skills, and Attitudes
for Advanced Practice Nursing Education (*continued*)

KNOWLEDGE	SKILLS	ATTITUDES
Examine strategies for improving systems to support team functioning	Engage in state and national policy initiatives aimed at improving teamwork and collaboration	

Note: Definition of teamwork and collaboration competency: Function effectively within nursing and interprofessional teams, fostering open communication, mutual respect, and shared decision making to achieve quality patient care.

Source: Reprinted from Cronenwett et al. (2009), with permission from Elsevier.

p. 25). Specific *Team and Teamwork (TT) Competencies* outlined in the report include:

TT1. Describe the process of team development and the roles and practices of effective teams.

TT2. Develop consensus on the ethical principles to guide all aspects of patient care and teamwork.

TT3. Engage other health professionals—appropriate to the specific care situation—in shared patient-centered problem solving.

TT4. Integrate the knowledge and experience of other professions—appropriate to the specific care situation—to inform care decisions, while respecting patient and community values and priorities/preferences for care.

TT5. Apply leadership practices that support collaborative practice and team effectiveness.

TT6. Engage self and others to constructively manage disagreements about values, roles, goals, and actions that arise among health care professionals and with patients and families.

TT7. Share accountability with other professions, patients, and communities for outcomes relevant to prevention and health care.

TT8. Reflect on individual and team performance for individual, as well as team, performance improvement.

TT9. Use process improvement strategies to increase the effectiveness of interprofessional teamwork and team-based care.

TT10. Use available evidence to inform effective teamwork and team-based practices.

TT11. Perform effectively on teams and in different team roles in a variety of settings. (IPEC, 2011, p. 25)

Source: Reprinted with permission of Association of American Medical Colleges (2011).

These teamwork competencies, along with the other interprofessional competencies in the report, have been designed to prepare all health professions students for "deliberatively working together with the common goal of building a safer and better patient-centered and community/population oriented US health care system" (IPEC, 2011, p. 25).

Analysis of all of the competencies posited by leadership groups in health care education further supports the common characteristics of teams discussed earlier, including mixed and complementary expertise, an agreed-upon common purpose, collective accountability and responsibility for outcomes, interdependence, collaboration, frank and open communication, conflict resolution, and shared decision making.

SUMMARY AND NEXT STEPS

This chapter began by asking you to look back on your life experiences as a member or leader of a team or partnership. Given what you now know about teams and partnerships, think again about those experiences. How often have you been a member of a team that was formed intentionally, choosing members based on expertise and complementary skills, who acted based on a common, stated purpose, with goals set for performance, a plan for how to accomplish those goals, and mutual accountability among members? How did your nursing education at all levels prepare you with the knowledge, skills, and competencies posited by nursing education leaders? How do you stack up against the team and teamwork competencies suggested by the IPEC Expert Panel? Simply identifying yourself as a member of a team, or calling a group a team, does not lead to effectiveness. The chapters that follow will help you to think about the elements that make a team effective, allowing you to build and lead strong teams and partnerships that have real impact on health care organizations and the people they serve.

QUESTIONS FOR THOUGHT

1. Describe a team in which you have been a member. How has the team demonstrated the common traits of teams as outlined in this chapter?

2. Imagine an ideal team in your organization. How might the common team traits of interdependence, collaboration, open and frank communication, and shared decision making be demonstrated in this team?

3. Compile a list of partnerships you know about in which your organization participates. How do these partnerships exemplify the common traits of partnerships such as collaboration, trust, equality, mutual understanding, and shared accountability? What would a partnership look like if these traits were not present?

4. Describe a situation you have experienced in which a team has impacted outcomes in a positive way? What characteristics or actions of that team affected the outcomes? Conversely, think about an experience in which the lack of teamwork led to a poor outcome? What opportunities by the team to make a positive impact were missed?

5. Think about how you were prepared to work as a team member or team leader in your nursing education. Describe those experiences that impacted your knowledge and skills about teamwork. How do your competencies as a team member or leader compare to those posited as essential competencies by organizations who are national leaders in nursing education? What skill gaps do you recognize as they relate to teaming?

6. Do you practice as a part of an interprofessional team? Does your team have the competencies outlined by the Interprofessional Education Collaboration (IPEC) as essential for interprofessional practice? If not, how will you develop those competencies?

TWO

Elements of Effective Nursing and Health Care Teams and Partnerships

A group becomes a team when each member is sure enough of himself and his contribution to praise the skill of the others.
—*Norman Shidle*

LEARNING OBJECTIVES

1. Discuss the importance of personal preferences related to teaming and partnering in selecting team members.
2. Describe the utility of three instruments used to assess personal preferences related to teamwork.
3. Analyze the potential impact of team champions, sponsors, and mentors on team effectiveness.
4. Apply the concept of collaborative capacity to teamwork in health care.
5. List 10 organizational factors that can lead to an increase in collaborative capacity.

Teams can only be as effective as their members. Therefore, selection of team members is an integral part of team effectiveness. The intentional selection of team members based on a series of key effectiveness factors will set up a team for success from inception. Remember that a team is made up of those with complementary skills. So, given the opportunity to select team members, team leaders should consider the individual preferences and tendencies of team members related to teaming and partnering, the ideal composition and balance of team member skills and competencies, relationships with team sponsors and mentors, the team climate, and the collaborative capacity of individuals when selecting a team.

PERSONAL PREFERENCES RELATED TO
TEAMING AND PARTNERING

Preferences are just that, a preferred way of operating in the world. Each of us has preferences, and each of us works within those preferences easily, but we can work outside of those preferences as well. Consider handedness; although we each have a preference for either our left or right hand, each of us uses both hands in our daily life. If we extend this analogy to other parts of our lives, for instance, our preferences for how we organize our life or our work, how we like to make decisions, how we process information, or how we choose to direct our energy, we can see how preferences may affect the work of a team. Successful team leaders will select teams that have a balance of preferences, and will use those preferences to support the work of the team. Although it is a temptation to select as partners those who have similar preferences to our own in work and life, in the case of effective teams, the team leader may be setting a team up for failure by not paying attention to diversity in individual preferences. Suppose for instance that you have selected a team in which everyone on the team processes information in the same way—they prefer to process information quickly, sometimes without thinking. These team members are impatient with long or slow tasks that require a lot of planning. Suppose your team task is to develop a community outreach program for vulnerable children in a culturally diverse neighborhood. How will this team succeed, processing information quickly without thought, with little appreciation for planning? Conversely, consider a team that is made up of all logical thinkers who prefer to make decisions based on data without attention to emotions or peoples' wishes. Place this team in the same situation. How will this team succeed at a task in which "data" may be lacking about logical solutions to the problem, and community relationships need to be considered? The team leader who has the opportunity will balance team member preferences and add diversity of thought and action to their team.

How then can you as a team leader understand the preferences of potential team members? First, your powers of observation will give you some insight into preferences. Every nurse leader can observe others around himself or herself, and has a fairly good assessment of how people prefer to work in groups. Observe others in meetings—are they quiet, contemplative, gregarious, or outgoing? Do they enjoy brainstorming in a group, or do they withdraw and come up with potential solutions alone or with a smaller group? Are they present-day thinkers, or do they look to the future? Do they enjoy organizing tasks? Do they confront conflict head on, or avoid it? Observant leaders can have a good picture of potential team members by studying individual behavior. However, for a more in-depth look at teaming preferences, team leaders can also use a variety of standardized tools, including the Myers–Briggs-Type Indicator (MBTI) and the Team Management Profile Questionnaire (TMPQ).

THE MYERS–BRIGGS-TYPE INDICATOR

The Myers–Briggs-Type Indicator is a useful method for understanding people that evaluates eight different personality preferences that individuals may use at different times. The eight preferences are organized into four opposite pairs, and the four preferences are combined into what the MBTI calls *types*. The MBTI has been used as a tool in a variety of industries, including government, small start-up companies and large global industries, education, and health care institutions (Hirsh & Kummerow, 1998). The MBTI can be used by individuals to gain a better understanding of the personal preferences and how they impact their work and life. Leaders can use his or her own MBTI to understand their preferences and gain insights into their leadership skills and areas of challenge. Team leaders can use the MBTI not only to understand their own behaviors but also to better appreciate other team members so as to make good use of individual differences, and approach problems in productive ways. Knowledge of type can help team leaders structure the team so as to have diversity of thought and action. In addition, the team leader can use his or her knowledge of type to develop creativity in teams, to help to resolve conflict, and to coach individual team members for success.

The MBTI was developed by Katharine Briggs and Isabel Myers, a mother-and-daughter team (Myers, McCaulley, Quenk, & Hammer, 1998). Their work on preference indicators is based on Jung's theory of psychological type. Over the past 50 years, thousands of studies have supported the use of the MBTI. In research evaluating the science and practice of team development, of the 176 respondents who listed psychological tests and/or assessment devices as a part of their team practice, a majority (55%) included the MBTI, making MBTI the most commonly used instrument in team development practice in this study (Offerman & Spiros, 2001). Thorson (2005) evaluated the effectiveness of the MBTI as a team-building tool. Thorson's study revealed that

50% of the participants in work teams were more confident in their ability to communicate with others, and that 60% felt their appreciation for different "types" within their team had changed as a result of using the MBTI tool. They also felt that improved self-awareness and ability to recognize individual differences enabled better communication, openness, and trust in the team.

MBTI Preferences

The four pairs of preferences in the MBTI are derived from four kinds of activities. These activities include how a person is energized (Extraversion or Introversion), what a person pays attention to (Sensing or Intuition), how a person makes decisions (Thinking or Feeling), and how a person chooses to live (Judging or Perceiving). Preferences in each of these activities have distinct characteristics as defined by Myers and Briggs (1998). For instance, in the *energizing* area, those who show preferences toward "extraversion" draw their energy from the outside world of people and activities, whereas those who tend toward the "introversion" preference draw their energy from their own internal world, including their own thoughts, ideas, and emotions. Contrary to popular conceptions, in the MBTI, extraversion and introversion have nothing to do with how gregarious, outgoing, talkative, or personable one is, but rather how one chooses to energize himself or herself. A very popular, engaging, and intellectual public speaker may prefer to leave a meeting and re-energize alone in her hotel room, rather than engage with others at postconference events. While using popular definitions, one would not think of someone who is an engaging public speaker as introverted, this example is the definition of *introversion* in MBTI language. The key is identification of where one draws energy. In the *perceiving* category, those who show preference toward "sensing" take in information through their senses and by noticing what is around them. Rather, those who show a preference on the other end of the dichotomy, "intuition," prefer to take in information through a "sixth sense," taking notice of the possibilities. A nurse leader who prefers to function following established procedures and standards alone would show preferences toward "sensing," whereas a leader who envisions the possibilities and innovative solutions to practical problems would likely show preferences toward "intuition." In the *deciding* category, those who show preference for organizing information in a logical manner would fall into the "thinking" category, and those who have a preference for organization of information based on their personal values would tend toward the "feeling" category. A team member who works systematically through problems using logic will likely show preferences toward thinking, whereas one who considers values, emotions, and seeks harmony would tend toward a feeling preference. Finally, in the *living* category, those who show preference for planning and organization in their life and work tend toward a "judging" preference, whereas those who are more spontaneous and open to new experiences are likely to tend toward a "perceiving" preference. Consider as an example the committee chairperson who seeks structure and scheduling of committee meetings, develops lists and agendas for meetings, and moves the committee toward closure rapidly, and contrast this to a committee chairperson who feels comfortable searching for options, allowing flexibility in meeting times and agenda, and re-visiting topics so as to include more information. These dichotomies would exemplify the working habits of those whose preferences were judging versus perceiving.

Upon completion of the MBTI questionnaire, participants receive a "score" on each of the dichotomies that places them into 1 of 16 types. Frequently, MBTI participants will use terms like "I'm a ENFJ," or "That's just the ISTP coming out in me." These types designate their composite in the areas of extraversion (E) versus introversion (I), sensing (S) versus intuition (N), thinking (T) versus feeling (F), and judging (J) versus perceiving (P). There are no good or bad types, and all preferences are valuable and necessary. Table 2.1 includes short descriptions of the 16 types.

Again, these types only indicate preferences, not skills or competencies. As with the example of handedness earlier, although we prefer to act as our type, we all have possibilities for expressing and using other characteristics as well. Leaders can find out more about the MBTI by visiting the Consulting Psychologists Press website at www.cpp.com. Multiple tools for application of the MBTI to teams, leadership, project management, decision making, and conflict can be found here.

So, how can the team leader use information gained from the MBTI to select teams with optimal composition for the task at hand? First, all perspectives are valuable to any organization. So, team leaders should strive to have diversity in types on the team. A balance of focus on the facts and the possibilities, structure, and free flow of ideas, logic, and emotions will enrich the work of any team. If one or more of the perspectives is missing, the team leader can seek to draw those preferences out of others in the team through creative techniques. Examples of using encouragement to tap into other preferences might be urging

TABLE 2.1
Short Descriptions of the 16 MBTI Types

ISTJ	ISFJ	INFJ	INTJ
Dependable	Accommodating	Compassionate	Analytical
Exacting	Detailed	Conceptual	Autonomous
Factual	Devoted	Creative	Determined
Logical	Loyal	Deep	Firm
Organized	Meticulous	Determined	Global
Practical	Organized	Idealistic	Independent
Realistic	Patient	Intense	Organized
Reliable	Practical	Intimate	Original
Reserved	Protective	Loyal	Private
Sensible	Quiet	Methodical	Systems minded
Steadfast	Responsible	Reflective	Theoretical
Thorough	Traditional	Sensitive	Visionary

ISTP	ISFP	INFP	INTP
Adaptable	Adaptable	Adaptable	Autonomous
Adventurous	Caring	Committed	Cognitive
Applied	Cooperative	Curious	Detached
Expedient	Gentle	Deep	Independent
Factual	Harmonious	Devoted	Logical
Independent	Loyal	Empathetic	Original
Logical	Modest	Gentle	Precise
Practical	Observant	Idealistic	Self-determined
Realistic	Sensitive	Imaginative	Skeptical
Resourceful	Spontaneous	Intimate	Speculative
Self-determined	Trusting	Loyal	Spontaneous
Spontaneous	Understanding	Reticent	Theoretical

ESTP	ESFP	ENFP	ENTP
Activity oriented	Adaptable	Creative	Adaptive
Adaptable	Casual	Curious	Analytical
Adventurous	Cooperative	Energetic	Challenging
Alert	Easygoing	Enthusiastic	Clever
Easygoing	Enthusiastic	Expressive	Enterprising
Energetic	Friendly	Friendly	Independent
Outgoing	Outgoing	Imaginative	Original
Persuasive	Playful	Independent	Outspoken
Pragmatic	Practical	Original	Questioning
Quick	Sociable	Restless	Resourceful
Spontaneous	Talkative	Spontaneous	Strategic
Versatile	Tolerant	Versatile	Theoretical

(continued)

TABLE 2.1
Short Descriptions of the 16 MBTI Types (*continued*)

ESTJ	ESFJ	ENFJ	ENTJ
Decisive	Conscientious	Appreciative	Challenging
Direct	Cooperative	Congenial	Controlled
Efficient	Harmonious	Diplomatic	Decisive
Gregarious	Loyal	Energetic	Energetic
Logical	Personable	Enthusiastic	Logical
Objective	Planful	Expressive	Methodical
Organized	Responsible	Idealistic	Objective
Practical	Responsive	Loyal	Opinionated
Responsible	Sociable	Organized	Planful
Structured	Sympathetic	Personable	Straightforward
Systematic	Tactful	Responsible	Strategic
Task focused	Traditional	Supportive	Tough minded

an ES, called by MBTI an "action-oriented realist," to try a creative approach rather than a practical approach to a problem, or encouraging an IS, called by MBTI a "thoughtful realist," to take an active role in a visioning exercise. Analysis of the team's preferences using a format as presented in Table 2.2 can be helpful for any team to consider how its preferences can be strengths and the potential pitfalls of those strengths as well.

Team leaders can systematically use information from the MBTI to craft a team development plan by looking at how the MBTI preferences might impact team relationships, skills, and processes. For instance, a team may want to consider MBTI preferences and their impact on how the team relates to one another, develops ground rules, or addresses conflict. Perhaps they may want to look at a skill inventory that will be helpful to their team's work, and how the preferences logically support those skills. The MBTI type may give clues as to who is comfortable with putting together complex reports, working under a deadline, or presenting ideas to a variety of stakeholder groups. Additionally, the MBTI types may help teams identify missing skill sets that will either need to be developed or added to the group. Finally, an understanding of the MBTI types of team members can help the group develop processes to support its work—using the balance of preferences to decide how meetings will occur or how communication is best structured in

TABLE 2.2
MBTI Team Analysis

Name	
My MBTI type	
Strengths of my type	1. 2. 3.
Potential weaknesses of my type	1. 2. 3.
MBTI of my teammates	**Type**
1. Name:	1.
2. Name:	2.
3. Name:	3.
MBTI team characteristics	1. 2. 3. 4.
Potential strengths of this team given the individual preference results?	1. 2. 3. 4.
Potential weaknesses of this team given the individual preference results?	1. 2. 3. 4.

the group. Using a form like that shown in Table 2.3 will aid a team in identifying goals supported by what they have learned in their MBTI exercises, and develop actions and responsibilities to support the team's future development.

Consider the following real-life team example using the MBTI. Think about the preferences that are missing in this team, and how the team leader could help the team's effectiveness through the development of other preferences in team members.

A team is developed to implement a nurse retention project in an intensive care unit at a large tertiary hospital. The turnover rate in the ICU has been unacceptably high. Team members include the nurse manager who is completing her Doctor of Nursing Practice degree, a new staff nurse, an experienced staff nurse who functions as a preceptor, and

TABLE 2.3
Team Development Plan

GOALS	ACTIONS	PERSON RESPONSIBLE	DATE DUE	RESOURCES NEEDED
Relationship goals				
1.				
2.				
3.				
Skills goals				
1.				
2.				
3.				
Process goals				
1.				
2.				
3.				

the director of staff development for the unit. The nurse manager is an ISTJ, who is thorough, systematic, hardworking, and careful with detail. She enjoys improvement of processes through facts and evidence, and is extremely loyal to the unit and organization. The new staff nurse is an ENFJ, who is interpersonally focused, tolerant, and has strong ideas about how the organization should treat others. The experienced staff nurse is an INTJ, who is independent, determined, and enjoys working by himself on complex projects. Finally, the staff development director is an INFP who is open-minded and flexible, and is constantly seeking new ideas to implement in the organization.

The nurse manager appoints the new staff nurse as leader of the team. How can this new nurse systematically use what she knows about the team to influence its success? What preferences will she need to encourage? Which preferences are missing and may need to be developed? Which are heavily represented and need to be used in some situations but may appear as weaknesses in other situations? How can the team use this information to craft a team development plan? The team leader uses a form like that in Table 2.2 to analyze the team using the MBTI. From this exercise, she and all team members can develop a plan for team development like the one in Table 2.3. The results for this team can be found in Table 2.4.

TABLE 2.4

Completed Team Analysis and Development Plan

Name	Staff nurse
My MBTI type	ENFJ
Strengths of my type	1. Enjoy leading and facilitating teams 2. Encourage cooperation 3. Participative stand in managing people and projects, challenge to make actions congruent with values
Potential weaknesses of my type	1. May ignore tasks and overly concentrate on relationships 2. May take criticism personally 3. May idealize others
MBTI of my team mates 1. Name: Nurse manager 2. Name: Experienced nurse 3. Name: Staff development director	Type 1. ISTJ 2. INTJ 3. INFP
MBTI team characteristics	1. Can be counted on to honor commitments 2. Draws individuals together with a common purpose 3. Strong ideas about the possible
Other team characteristics	1. Nurse manager completing her DNP, understands systems-level change 2. Preceptor expertise present in experienced staff nurse team member 3. Staff development has active network of other hospital-based educators for benchmarking
Potential strengths of this team given the individual preference results?	1. Work together to remove obstacles and achieve the possible 2. Organizational loyalty 3. Communicative and persuasive 4. Facilitative

TEAM DEVELOPMENT PLAN

GOALS	ACTIONS	PERSON RESPONSIBLE	DATE DUE	RESOURCES NEEDED
Relationship goal:				
Provide everyone with an opportunity to talk (E vs. I)	Team leader (E) will consciously seek input during meetings from all team members	Team leader	First meeting and ongoing	May need meeting facilitation guidelines or training for team leader Team ground rules to include seeking input from all during meeting
Skills goal:				
Develop conflict management skills	Develop ground rules and model for conflict resolution at outset of team meeting	Team	First team meeting	Conflict resolution model and training
	Adhere to ground rules at all meetings and in all interactions		All team meetings	
Integrate inherent skills of group into project development and management (systems-level change knowledge, preceptor experience, etc.)	Encourage participation of all in project development	Team leader and team	All team meetings	

(continued)

31

TABLE 2.4
Completed Team Analysis and Development Plan (*continued*)

| | TEAM DEVELOPMENT PLAN | | | |
GOALS	ACTIONS	PERSON RESPONSIBLE	DATE DUE	RESOURCES NEEDED
	Consider strengths of individuals in assigning responsibilities			Presentation on system level change by nurse manager Presentation on current preceptor system by Staff Development officer and experienced nurse/preceptor
Process goal: Balance vision with facts, organization with flexibility.	Develop team mechanisms for balanced views through team processes. Allow for presentations of facts, along with visioning/what is possible exercises	Team leader and team	All team meetings	Stakeholders in problem to present data/facts (e.g., Human Resources (HR), Quality Improvement (QI), etc.) Benchmark data on how other organizations have designed programs to decrease attrition from ICU Facilitator for visioning exercises

Crafting a team development plan in this case allows all team members to participate in the identification of strengths and weaknesses, and facilitates all team members' understanding the direction of the team. Purposeful actions like taking the time to understand the team and developing a team development plan are what separates effective teams from those fraught with conflict, indecision, and inability to complete tasks.

THE TEAM MANAGEMENT PROFILE QUESTIONNAIRE

Another useful tool for the team to use in understanding its preferences, skills, and competencies is the Team Management Profile Questionnaire (TMPQ). Team Management Systems' TMPQ (www.tms.com.au) is an assessment that is used as part of a model describing the dynamics of high-performing teams (McCann, 2009). McCann (2003) includes the TMPQ as part of the Workplace Behavior Pyramid, which includes assessments of values, risk orientation, and preferences (Figure 2.1).

McCann developed this model to assist leaders in developing effective teams, motivating team members with assigned tasks, and delivering excellent outcomes. The model provides us with a picture of how people approach their work (McCann, 2003).

The base of the Work Behavior Pyramid as developed by McCann is values. McCann defines *values* as "fundamental concepts or beliefs which people use to guide their behavior in the workplace" (McCann, 2009, p. 7). Values influence all aspects of our work and professional lives, including decision making, conflicts, and our view of people and the organization. Values can energize people around causes that threaten their beliefs; likewise, most people support actions that are in concert with their values. Although evaluation of values is difficult, McCann (2009) has developed the Window on Work Values, a 64-item questionnaire that describes activities in the workplace that the participant values. Teams can use the Window on Work Values scale to develop a profile of team values and plan their work to reinforce those values.

McCann adds the analysis of risk orientation to the middle of the model of workplace behavior. Risk orientation, according to McCann, is an analysis of the tendencies of individuals to see opportunities versus see obstacles. McCann has developed the Opportunities–Obstacle Quotient ($QO2^R$) to analyze an individual's approach to risk. This scale has five subscales, all relating to risk orientation. These subscales, including *moving toward goals, multi-pathways, time focus, fault finding,* and *optimism* may help to predict behavior in team situations. Risk

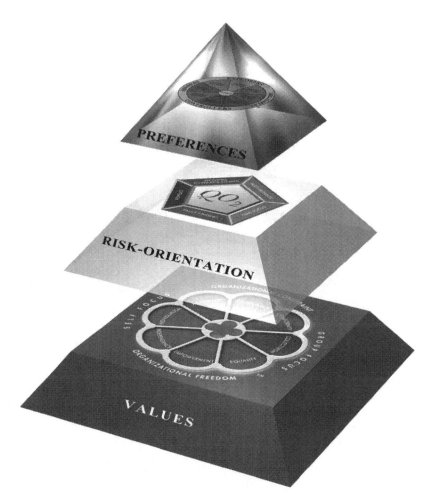

FIGURE 2.1 McCann pyramid of workplace behavior.
Source: Reproduced by permission of Dr. Dick McCann,
Team Management Systems, www.tms.com.au.

orientation can certainly affect the work of a group and may have a cumulative effect with individual preferences. The risk orientation tendencies of a team may influence a team's ability to see the possibilities versus giving up. A balance of risk orientation is valuable to a team.

At the very top of the model is work preferences. McCann and colleagues developed the TMPQ to understand an individual's approaches to work. After completing the questionnaire, participants are provided with a personal Team Management Profile, developed to provide constructive information outlining work preferences and the strengths that an individual brings to a team. Work preferences are explored in the areas of *relationships, information gathering and use, decision making,* and *organization.* The personal Team Management Profile highlights an individual's major and related areas of work preferences, with a focus on individual and leadership strengths, decision making, interpersonal skills, and team building. The report provides the participants with areas for self-assessment, which allows team members to develop action plans and improve team performance. Information in the report can also help team members understand how best to communicate with one another.

TEAM CLIMATE

The climate within which a team's activities occur can be as integral to a team's effectiveness as any other factor. Team climate has been defined by Anderson and West (1998) as a team's shared perceptions of organizational policies, practices, and procedures. In developing their Team Climate Inventory (Anderson & West, 1998), they used a four-factor theory developed previously in research into climate and innovation (West, 1990). The four factors their instrument is based upon are *vision, participative safety, task orientation,* and *support for innovation.*

Vision in the context of team climate refers to the idea that the team holds about the valued outcome of their work, and a motivational force for their work. The vision must be understandable, valued by the group, widely accepted among the team members, and reasonably attainable through the group's work. The presence of team vision therefore is an integral factor in team climate. *Participative safety* is a concept that refers to the nonthreatening nature of the team that impacts its functioning. Participative safety exists when any member of the team feels able to propose ideas, problems, and solutions in a nonthreatening environment. *Task orientation* refers to a commitment among team members to excellence in performance of tasks. It is evidenced by emphasis on accountability, systems for evaluating and modifying performance, reflection on performance among team members, feedback, and cooperation. Finally, *support for innovation* is the degree to which either implicit or explicit support exists for finding new ways to do the work of the team. Consider the following case while applying West's four factors to your thinking about the team climate.

> The leadership team at a local branch of a large long-term care organization consists of the chief executive officer (CEO), the chief operations officer (COO), the chief financial

officer (CFO), and the chief nursing officer (CNO). The CNO also serves as the chief quality and safety officer for the organization. The CEO is known as a visionary leader, and the team has agreed to the vision of the organization which mirrors the corporate vision of "improving the quality of life of everyone we serve." As a visionary, the CEO thinks of *himself* as a "big picture thinker," and allows the rest of the team to take care of the details. The chief operations officer is the face of the organization, and does most of the talking at meetings. She is conflict averse, and so therefore sees team meetings as informational, but not as times to problem solve. She sees her role as assuring that all operations at the local site are carried out in exactly the same way as they are dictated by the parent organization, and in the same way that they are carried out in all of the other local organizations. The CFO is constantly concerned about the bottom line, and is also concerned that personnel costs are being kept artificially low, and that this may have an impact on keeping a skilled workforce. The CNO is brand new to her role, and is observing the team at work.

What could the CNO learn about the team climate for this team, and how can she use it to the best advantage of her team of providers who are on the front lines of care? First, the vision of the organization seems to be explicitly accepted by the organization. However, do the actions of the team support that vision? Concerns about a skilled workforce may have direct impact on the team realizing that vision. So, are there implicit factors in the climate that are undermining the vision? Next, what has the CNO learned about participative safety? On first glance, it sounds as if this team may be threatened if they speak up about issues. The CNO will need to further explore this segment of team climate in order to assure herself that she will be safe to discuss problems in the team. Has she learned anything about task orientation? She has likely learned little about commitment to excellence in this team, and will need to further assess the climate as she continues to work with the team. Finally, she likely assumes that support for innovation is low in this organization, as the parent organization is dictating action. However, she notes that she will need to assess the ability of the team to impact the decisions of the parent organization.

Simple observations can allow team leaders and members to assess the potential impact of climate factors on their team's effectiveness.

Being aware of the impact of team climate helps leaders to develop strategies to build a climate that is supportive of the team's work.

TEAM CHAMPIONS, SPONSORS, AND MENTORS

Just as integral to selecting team members with personal preferences toward teaming and partnerships for team effectiveness is the notion of developing successful relationships with team champions, sponsors, and mentors. Just as the work of the team members can impact the effectiveness of the team, so can the work of these other external team supporters. Let us examine the important team roles of *champion, sponsor,* and *mentor* that can impact team success.

A *team champion* is usually considered to be the person outside of the team who takes responsibility for pushing a team's work forward, gathering resources and support from people, teams, and other departments in an organization. Without a team champion, the chances of success are diminished. The team champion invests in the team's success, as the champion typically has personal involvement and a stake in the success of the team's work. Consider the example below and think about the actions of the team champion that can potentially lead to the team's success.

> Three county health departments have come together to partner across their agencies to develop and implement plans for mass rapid immunization against an emerging influenza virus. The decision was made to partner across these politically disparate organizations as they are all small departments with limited staff, have immense but similar needs, and are close in geographic location, in fact, their county borders are contiguous. The three lead nurses from each of the three county health departments, as well as the three county health officers, are the team members. The idea for this partnership was born by the state health officer, who has stated that his vision is to make working to develop collaborative relationships across health departments the norm, and sees this as a pilot for future programs. The team is selected by the state health officer, given their charge, and begins work on developing their plan. In developing their plan, they develop outcome criteria, monthly goals, and identify key resources needed, including access to vaccine in an expedited time period, funding for vaccine clinics, additional

temporary staff to support the rapid immunization plan, and assistance in public relations in their county. Although not directly involved in the planning or implementation of the program, the state health officer uses his contacts at the vaccine clearinghouse to allow for rapid access to vaccine, makes a request to the governor for additional short-term funding of vaccine clinics including a temporary workforce, and makes this project a priority for his chief of public relations to quickly develop a multimedia campaign for the three affected counties. The team implements the plan and evaluates success against their desired outcomes. The team champion uses those outcomes in public addresses and with the governor and legislature as a demonstration of how collaboration across agencies can impact team success.

What actions of the *team champion* led to the effectiveness of this team? First, the team champion in this scenario had a stake in the team's success—the state health officer has interest in the success of this team, because he wants to use the successful collaboration demonstrated here as a stepping stone to successful collaboration in other cross-agency partnerships—part of his vision for the state public health organization. Next, he garners resources that he can access more easily than the team can to assure their success—for instance, funding from the Governor for the pilot project. Although the team perhaps could have worked to garner similar resources from other sources, the team champion can quickly develop buy-in for the project at high levels of state government, which may be helpful in future projects. Finally, the team champion makes the team's process a priority for related players external to the team, further influencing the success of the team. As is demonstrated here, team champions can be invaluable to the success of a team, and the team is wise to find champions and to build relationships with those champions during their work together.

A *team sponsor* may or may not be the same as the champion. The sponsor is not a team member but supports the team, helps to gain resources for it, and works to clear obstacles from its path. The sponsor usually has a deeper understanding of the organization, its culture, climate, and politics than individual team members may have. The sponsor will typically meet with the team periodically throughout their process to help them to identify pathways within an organization to facilitate the team's success, and to help identify and plan for removal of barriers to success. Usually, the sponsor is from a higher level of management, allowing insights into potential pathways for team success, and access to upper management for assistance. Consider the following example of the importance of a sponsor in a team's success.

> A team of intensive care nurses from across a large tertiary hospital come together to discuss methods to increase retention of new graduate nurses in the intensive care unit (ICU). Turnover in the first year of employment for new graduates is now 33% in the ICU, which leads to increased costs of replacement, decreased staff morale, and potentially lower quality care. The team, made up of nurses from four different ICUs across the hospital, is led by a nurse who has been exploring the evidence surrounding the impact of nurse residency programs in decreasing nurse turnover rates as part of her DNP program. The team comes together to discuss implementation of a nurse residency program in the organization, and quickly realizes that a number of organizational approvals and perhaps barriers may exist, and that their expertise does not extend to the broader organization. They identify the director of nursing Recruitment and Retention as their team sponsor. This nurse reports directly to the chief nursing officer, and has been with the organization for 25 years. The team sponsor meets with the team, thinks that their plan is sound, and helps them to identify how to move this project through the organizational approval process while looking at potential barriers and solutions to overcome those barriers. The team sponsor helps the team to develop a plan for presenting the plan to the ICU committee, to the Nursing Education Council, and to the CNO. The sponsor helps the team to think through possible arguments against the project (funding, acceptance, human resources issues, staffing, etc.), and possible solutions (grant funding, public relations, education, piloting the program to analyze impact on staffing, etc.) to present to the various stakeholders to avoid those barriers leading to program failure. The team works to move the project through the organizational approvals, and continues to work together through implementation and evaluation of the project. The team sponsor continues to meet with the team to help identify ways to publicize the results of the project both within and outside of the organization, and to work to implement the program in additional areas of high turnover.

In this case example, how did the work of the sponsor differ from the work of the champion in the first example? In this example, the team sponsor provides expertise to the team in moving their work forward in the organization, but does not necessarily garner resources or buy-in for the project using their own influence, rather the sponsor teaches the team how to succeed. In the first example, the team champion used their influence to directly impact the success of the team through providing the appropriate resources and support. As you can see, depending on the situation, either or both of these roles external to the team may influence the team's success.

A *team mentor* is quite different than a champion or sponsor. The team mentor usually has specific expertise in the area of team interest. A mentor should have a breadth of experience in an area of the team's work so that she can effectively discuss technical issues with team members and refer them to appropriate resources to gain more knowledge in a particular area of interest. A mentor can answer team members' questions, discuss issues they raise, and suggest resources for problem solving. However, the mentor does not usually use her influence to solve problems that the team confronts, nor to bring to bear any resources to impact the team's success. Consider the following example of a team mentor, and how this team makes use of the mentor's expertise for team success.

> A team of nursing faculty members is interested in using social media to recruit students to an online postgraduate certificate program in nursing ethics. Although the faculty members have combined expertise in online education, nursing curriculum development, and the content area of nursing ethics, they have little expertise in the use of social media as a recruitment tool. One team member brings to a team meeting an example of how her child's high school has begun using social media to recruit students for community service activities. The effort is innovative, using a combination of a variety of social media methods and sites for recruitment, and is led by a parent who has expertise in public relations and social media campaigns through his work with a local nonprofit. The faculty team invites the parent to dinner with the team and spends about 2 hours asking targeted questions about his experience with different social media methods, reaching out to professionals using social media, the elements of successful social media

campaigns for different age groups, the requirements for hardware and software, and the ongoing management of a social media campaign. The mentor is able to share his expertise and refer the team to a variety of additional resources to broaden their understanding of the use of social media for recruitment. Finally, the mentor is able to link the team to other local experts in the community who they can work with to successfully implement their campaign. The team applies this newfound understanding and expertise to develop a social media campaign to recruit for their program, which progresses as their knowledge and experience broadens.

Different then from the champion and sponsor who use their influence and expertise to directly impact the success of the team, the mentor has a more indirect role in sharing knowledge with the team, and linking the team to expertise in an area where they are lacking. The team then can apply that expertise to their particular goals. Mentors can bring strength to a team in ways that champions and sponsors may not, allowing new knowledge to be applied to the team's work.

COLLABORATIVE CAPACITY

For any team or partnership to make use of all the skills and roles discussed in this chapter, their individual collaborative capacity as well as the collaborative capacity of the organization must be finely tuned. Individual collaborative capacity can be defined as the knowledge, skills, and attitudes required to achieve collaborative outcomes (Carrasco, 2009). Organizational collaborative capacity can be defined as the culture and processes required to support collaboration (Carrasco, 2009). The capacity to collaborate cannot be forced, merely assigning a team does not create collaborative capacity. Rather, there must be an inherent wish to collaborate, supported by knowledge, skills, and attitudes that facilitate working with others to achieve common goals. Hence, team leaders will be wise to analyze potential team members for these traits using some of the tools identified in this chapter.

Although part of this capacity comes from within the individual team member, collaborative capacity is also facilitated by the organization. According to Erickson (2009), organizations must create environments that encourage people to "become engaged, to take initiative, invest discretionary effort in a wide variety of collaborative activities, and, as a result, develop new approaches and ideas for their work" (p. 1). Erickson implores organizational leaders to think of the challenge "as one of setting the stage, creating an environment that engages players from multiple constituencies" (p. 1).

Erickson's team has identified 10 organizational factors that lead to an increase in individual and organizational collaborative capacity. They include:

1. Highly engaged, committed participants
2. Trust-based relationships
3. Prevalence of networking opportunities
4. Collaborative hiring, development, and promotion practices
5. Organizational philosophy supporting "community of adults"
6. Leaders with both task- and relationship-management skills
7. Executive role models for collaboration
8. Productive and efficient behaviors and processes
9. Well-defined individual roles and responsibilities
10. Important, challenging tasks

Organizational leaders can set their teams up for success by attending to these factors in their organizational culture, climate, and philosophy. More strategies around this topic can be found in Chapter 5.

SUMMARY AND NEXT STEPS

Teams can only be as effective as their members. Purposeful selection of team members is integral for team effectiveness. The tools provided in this chapter help leaders with the intentional selection of team members based on a series of key effectiveness factors. When team leaders have the opportunity to select their own teams, consideration of the individual preferences and tendencies of team members related to teaming and partnering, the ideal composition and balance of team member skills and competencies, relationships with team sponsors and mentors, the team climate, and the collaborative capacity of individuals when selecting a team will only enhance the team's performance. In future chapters, the characteristics of teams will be revisited as we consider ways that leaders can maximize their functioning.

QUESTIONS FOR THOUGHT

1. As a team leader, you have an opportunity to select team members for an upcoming project in your organization. How would you approach the selection of your team?
2. Consider how you might use any of the team preference analyses in this chapter in team selection.
3. Think about a current team of which you are a member. Do you have a team champion? What does that team champion assist the team to accomplish? If you do not have a team champion, how could a team champion improve your work?
4. Analyze the differences among team champions, sponsors, and mentors. How does each potentially impact the success of a team? Could the same person serve in all roles with a team? If so, how might their effectiveness be impacted?

THREE

Getting Started: Building a Strong Team

A team is more than a collection of people. It is a process of give and take.
—Barbara Glacel and Emile Robert, Jr.

LEARNING OBJECTIVES

1. Discuss the advantages of building a team based on diverse strengths.
2. Analyze the four domains of leadership strengths present in effective teams.
3. Understand methods for gathering data about team member skills and team strengths.
4. Use observational techniques for skills analysis.
5. Apply formal skills analysis techniques in team formation.
6. Identify methods to analyze skill gaps and to develop plans to fill those gaps.

If teams are truly the sum of their parts, then building a strong team will take work to put all of the right parts in place. This process takes the time, energy, and insight of the leader and team members to assure that the right people are in the right positions within the team in order to meet goals. Regardless of whether the team is a naturally occurring team, or one that has been selected for a particular purpose, building a strong team will require an analysis of skills and strengths, planning for application of those skills and strengths, and thoughtful consideration of how to fill skill gaps. Peter Drucker, sometimes called the "inventor of modern management," once said, "Unless, therefore, an executive looks for strength and works at making strength productive, he will only get the impact of what a man cannot do, of his lacks, his weaknesses, his impediments to performance and effectiveness. To staff from what there is not and to focus on weakness is wasteful—a misuse, if not abuse, of the human resource" (Drucker, 2007, p. 80). Team leaders should heed these words, and consider how to build on strengths as they build their teams.

In Chapter 2, we discussed preferences related to teamwork and teaming. A variety of teamwork preference assessments were suggested, and ideas for how to use these in team development were presented. In this chapter, we will look at how these preferences can be translated by leaders into actions to build the strongest team possible. In their book *Strengths Based Leadership*, Rath and Conchie point out that the most effective leaders surround themselves with the right people and then maximize their team. They posit that although the best leaders are not well-rounded, the best teams are. Rath and Conchie have found that strong, cohesive teams have a representation of strengths in four domains—executing, influencing, relationship building, and strategic thinking (2009). These four domains of leadership strength are critical to the overall effective functioning of a team. Team members who have a dominant strength in the *Executing* domain are those whom the team depends upon to implement a solution. These are the people who will work to accomplish the goal. Team members who are strong in the *Executing* domain are skilled in taking an idea and transforming it into reality. People who are skilled at *Influencing* can be counted on by the team to sell the team's ideas inside and outside the organization. The team member with the talent to take charge, speak up, and make sure the group is heard is one who is skilled in the domain of *Influencing*.

Relationship builders pull and hold a team together. Strengths associated with bringing people together in a variety of ways transform a group of individuals into a team moving with a common purpose. *Strategic thinkers* are those who are skilled at keeping their team focused on the possible, and are constantly pulling a team and its members into the future. They absorb, analyze, and translate information that will assist the team to make the right decisions to meet its goals.

INDIVIDUAL TALENTS, SKILLS, AND TEAM STRENGTH ANALYSIS

Any team needs to play from the strength of its members. Consider a baseball team with a strong pitcher and a not so strong outfield. However, the outfielders are successful hitters with the highest batting averages on the team. This team's strategy should always be to play from their position of strength—to get as many strikeouts as possible, to try to avoid pitches that will result in hard hits to the outfield, and to get as many players on base as possible before their outfielders are at bat—so that they can drive in runs. Team leaders for this team have objective data or "team statistics" upon which to base their analysis of skills and strengths. Batting averages, runs batted in, strikeouts, earned run averages, and errors make up their assessment of individual skills and team strengths. Their game plan is driven by this knowledge. But how does this translate into a game plan for a health care team?

The first step in developing a game plan for your team will be to consider how you will gather data about talents, skills, and strengths. There are a number of informal and formal methods you can use to gather your "team stats." These include self-analysis and report, observation during team tasks, and formal skills assessments.

Self-Analysis and Report

Introspection will help team members to understand themselves and the talents and skills that they can offer a team. Prior to joining a team, team members should be encouraged to think about their talents and skills and share those up front with the team leader and team members. Particular talents and skills that might be important to a team include ability to strategize, coaching skills, creativity, communication acumen, dealing with conflict, judgment, open mindedness, and bridge building. Other teams may need specific skills related to their mission, like ability to manage data, writing and presentation skills, or powers of persuasion. Team members who can quickly identify their talents and skills and share them openly with the team will facilitate the building of the team's strength.

Consider, for example, a recent doctor of nursing practice (DNP) graduate who is being recruited to join an interprofessional team working to develop a statewide smoking cessation program for pregnant women to be implemented in clinics, hospitals, and private practices during the prenatal period. An evidence-based protocol has been adopted, and the challenge of the team will be to coordinate efforts among multiple agencies to establish reimbursement for the intervention; to roll out the intervention in unique ways for different organizations, cultures, and populations; to make the change "stick"; and to evaluate the impact of the intervention. Clearly, DNP graduates are prepared with competencies related to evidence-based practice, population health, leadership, teamwork, and health policy, so the competencies needed to succeed with this work should be there. But how can the DNP graduate prepare to articulate the particular skills that she brings to the team during the interview process? Questions that the nurse might ask to pinpoint the skill set she possesses that could be of value to the team include:

- Where do I fit in when I work in a team? What is my typical role when I work in groups? What do I like to do when I am a member of a team?
- Do I cooperate with others, lead, follow, guide, advise, coach, strategize, create?
- Do I prefer the big picture, or am I a detail person?
- Do I like to be the recorder in a team meeting?
- Are there times when I tend to take a more active role? What is happening to make me take a more active role? What are the conditions that are present that facilitate my active participation?
- Do I like to be the spokesperson for a group? Am I a good public speaker?
- How do I handle conflict? Am I a peacekeeper? A negotiator? Do I shy away from conflict?
- How does my personality impact my work in a team? Do I tend to dominate? Or do I tend to allow others to talk, and I listen? Can I help the group to distinguish between the important and trivial?
- Am I an idea person? Do I share my ideas readily? Do I like to build on ideas of others?

It becomes obvious that the value of this member to the team will be strengthened with the answers to some of these questions. Consider the difference between a potential team member who says, "I learned about change, leadership, and evidence-based practice in my DNP program," and the interviewee who comes equipped with the answers to the questions above, and shares with the interviewer that "My role in teams is typically as a strategizer, a problem solver, and a negotiator. I have been called upon by teammates to help us come up with multiple solutions to particular problems, and to guide us toward consensus around the best possible strategy given our situation. I usually serve as the spokesperson for groups, as I am able to articulate ideas clearly and energetically. I am not great with managing large data sets, and prefer to allow those who are good at this to take the lead in this area." This response shows personal insight, an understanding of talents and strengths that can benefit the team, and recognition of how the strengths of others can also benefit the team. Sharing these specific insights allows the team to see exactly where this member could fit. These two responses demonstrate the difference between an introspective team member and one who has not taken the time to evaluate her own strengths that can be integral to team success.

Observational Methods of Strength Analysis

Team leaders can learn a lot about their current or potential team members through observation of their work, and through purposeful interview of team members or candidates. Although it might be easy to observe someone's technical skills, identifying someone's interpersonal skills and strengths takes more effort.

The following tips were adapted from those developed by the Mindtools organization (MindTools, n.d.) to help to assess current or future team members for appropriateness to the team.

Listen carefully: For example, when you ask a job candidate to explain the best moment at her last job, listen closely. If she talks about when she influenced a key decision, she might be skilled in influencing, interpersonal relationships, and strategy. A good question might be if she ever served on a committee or executive board, and how she used her skills in that role. When you are working with a potential team member, listen to how she interacts with others on the team. Is she is empathic, strategic, analytical? Consider how these skills that you observe will mesh with those of your team, and how these strengths can propel your team forward with its mission.

Structure your conversation around a specific skill: For instance, if you need to find a new team member who is strong in interpersonal skills, observe how he interacts in a natural workgroup, or structure your interview around that skill. You could ask the candidate to describe how he would resolve a conflict between two other colleagues. You could even try role playing or provide a real-life example from your team, and ask him how he would approach the problem if he were a team member.

Notice how the person makes you feel: Pay attention to how you feel when talking to the potential team member, and observe how that person interacts with other members of the team. If he gets people excited and motivated about their work, or about the opportunities that the organization faces, then he might excel at team leadership. If he is inquisitive and always posing the important questions for the team, he might be a natural team member to facilitate brainstorming and "what-if" forecasting.

Formal Skills Assessments

Individual Analysis

More formal methods of self-evaluation may also be useful to teams. One popular method of self-evaluation for team members is a series of assessments developed over the last 15 years by Tom Rath (2007) through his work with the "father of strengths psychology" Donald O. Clifton and the Gallup Organization (p. i). Based on 40 years of studying strengths in humans, a list of the 34 most common talents was developed, and these became the basis of the Clifton StrengthsFinder Assessment. The purpose of the assessment was to assist people to discover their strengths and to be able to describe their talents. The Gallup Organization's own surveys of over 10 million people found that only about one-third of people strongly agree with the statement "At work, I have the opportunity to do what I do best every day." Although this is a concerning finding, fortunately, Gallup research found that when people do have the opportunity to focus on their strengths, they are six times as likely to be engaged in their jobs, and more than three times as likely to report an excellent quality of life (p. iii). In 2007, Rath released the StrengthsFinder 2.0 assessment in his book by the same name. For those who purchase the book, an online assessment provides not only an opportunity for team members to discover their strengths, but also an action planning guide based on the unique strengths of each team member. The 34 strengths included in the StrengthsFinder 2.0 cover the gamut of human talents, and range from activator (one who has a talent for taking action that can make things happen), to includer (one who wants to expand groups so that as many people as possible can benefit), to relator (one who has a talent for deep and genuine relationships). Through discovering areas of talent in a team, a team leader can manage those talents, and can identify and manage areas of lesser talent as well as blind spots, described by Rath as times when our talents derail our pursuits (p. 24).

Consider the team who is challenged to transform the culture of a free clinic from one of task orientation to one of patient-centered services. The team leader understands that cultural transformations can be derailed by a number of factors, including among others a lack of ownership of the change, a lack of leadership, outside forces, and diverse cultures within the organization (Scott, Mannion, Davies, & Marshall, 2003a, 2003b). In this clinic, the task-oriented culture is necessary because of scarce resources, and has been dominated by a strong paraprofessional workforce. However, a recent audit of the clinic's patient outcomes, including satisfaction, has indicated that return visits are few, patients do not perceive having a strong relationship to the clinic, and that patients overwhelmingly express feeling as if they are treated as a "number." The Board of Trustees has asked the chief executive officer (CEO) to lead a transformation of the culture to be more consistent with the vision and mission of the organization, which has always been to "provide compassionate care to the whole person regardless of ability to pay." The CEO decides to appoint a team and leader to work on this cultural transformation, but first elects to use a StrengthsFinder 2.0 assessment to help to build the team.

The profile of employees who are selected for the team is shown in Table 3.1. The team leader must develop a plan to use the strengths of the team in appropriate ways to facilitate change. How do you think the leader could make best use of the skills of these team members?

Consider how the team leader can plan to best use the strengths and talents of each team member in his or her work. For example, who might be the best person on the team to lead brainstorming? To analyze data? To remember the past? To facilitate goal setting? To partner with and bring along internal groups? To work with external forces? To see through the plans? To resolve conflicts? To serve as "cheerleader"? To evaluate the impact? Through this brief exercise, it becomes clear that team members have a variety of talents that can facilitate the team's success, and these strengths are not related necessarily to their level of professional achievement, education, or position within the organization. Rather, the team leader, through working with the team's strengths and talents, instead of other preconceived notions of the value of team members, can facilitate the success of the team, and ultimately the transformation of the culture of the organization. The leader can put every member in a position in which they can call on their strengths and contribute the most to the team and the project. So, while the strength of each team member is important, it is more important to put together a team that is strong because of the talents of its members.

Team Analysis

Other methods of skill and strengths analysis involve the input of the entire team. Team Management Systems (TMS) has highlighted the common elements responsible for integrating and coordinating teams into a coherent "whole" through interviews with teams and leaders from around the world. TMS (www/tms.com.au/linkingskills.html) identifies these elements as *Linking Skills*. According to TMS, research has shown that it is difficult for an individual to assess his or her own "skills" accurately. A person can only be considered to have Linking

TABLE 3.1
Team Strengths Using StrengthsFinder 2.0

TEAM MEMBER	TOP TWO STRENGTHS	BRIEF DESCRIPTION OF STRENGTHS
Nurse manager (team leader)	Achiever Empathy	Constant need for achievement Sees the world through other's eyes; senses the emotions of others
Physician/ medical director	Analytical Self-assurance	Objective, dispassionate, data driven Faith in own strengths, able to deliver
Lead medical assistant	Positivity Woo (Winning Others Over)	Always finds positivity in any situation Enjoys the challenge of meeting new people, energized by strangers
Lab technician	Individualization Maximizer	Intrigued by the unique qualities of each person Seeks out and nurtures strengths
Pharmacist	Ideation Responsibility	Fascinated by ideas, always looking for connections, new perspectives Takes psychological ownership of any commitment
Reception clerk	Focus Relator	Goals serve as compass, evaluates whether particular actions will lead to a goal Derives strengths from genuine relationships, encourages deepening of relationships
Consumer of services (patient)	Context Harmony	Looks back to understand the present Looks for areas of agreement, little is gained from conflict and friction, works to hold these to a minimum

Source: Rath (2007).

Skills if he or she is recognized as such by others who interact with the person concerned on a regular basis. TMS's three Linking Skills Profile Questionnaires are multirater assessments through which a number of different people rate an individual's linking skills. The Linking of People Profile Questionnaire is used for all team members and gives feedback on the six people linking skills identified by TMS. These people linking skills include active listening, communication, team relationships, problem solving and counseling, participative decision making, and interface management. The Linking of People and Tasks Profile Questionnaire is used for senior team members and gives feedback on six People Linking Skills plus five Task Linking Skills. Task

Linking Skills include objective setting, quality standards, work allocation, team development, and delegation. The Linking Leader Profile Questionnaire is ideal for team leaders and addresses three sets of Linking Skills, including People Linking Skills, Task Linking Skills, and Leadership Linking Skills. The additional Leadership Linking Skills included in this profile include motivation and strategy. Ideally, Linking Skills Profile Questionnaires are completed by the self, direct reports, peers, and managers. Respondents to the questionnaires assess the extent to which the Linking Skill *should occur*, and the importance of the particular skill in the work of the team. The rater is then asked to assess the individual in terms of what actually does occur. The Linking Skills Profiles assess the gap between what *should occur* and what *does occur* and is reported as rates of satisfaction. A graphic colored summary of the importance and satisfaction rates is presented for each Linking Skill, along with key advice generated from the response by the raters to each question. A quantitative report offers a detailed analysis of each Linking Skill. Team leaders and members may find this type of formal self- and team assessment to be extremely helpful in assessing the strength of the team. The results of the questionnaires can enable the individual to develop focused action plans to improve linking or for the team to identify who on the team is best suited to a variety of tasks.

Another formal profile that has been developed to analyze specific strengths of individual health care team members is the Communication and Teamwork Skills (CATS) assessment (Frankel, Gardner, Maynard, & Kelly, 2007). The CATS assessment is a behavior-based tool that is based on principles of crisis resource management used in nonmedical industries. The CATS Assessment was developed to quantitatively assess communication and team skills of health care providers in a variety of real and simulated clinical settings. The CATS Assessment has been developed through rapid-cycle improvement and tested through observation of videotaped simulated clinical scenarios, real-time surgical procedures, and multidisciplinary rounds. Specific behaviors assessed by the CATS include coordination, cooperation, situational awareness, and communication. Team members are scored in terms of the occurrence and quality of the behaviors. Reports allow health care providers to view an overall score for the categories as well as scores for specific behaviors. Although this tool has been developed for use with clinical teams providing direct patient care, elements of the team's behavior are translatable to a variety of team situations. For instance, in assessing the behavior of coordination, elements such as team briefings and de-briefing and verbalizing a plan with expected time frames are observed. These behaviors are essential for team success in a variety of team circumstances. Likewise, in the area of communication, elements of teamwork assessed, including verbal updates of plan, closed-loop communication, and appropriate tone of voice during communication, are equally as important in any teamwork situation.

SKILL GAPS

Team leaders strive to facilitate the highest performance of all members of the team given the strengths of each individual member and the power that comes from combining those skills in a team. However, even with the best planning, a team and team leader may note that skill gaps exist. Just like the baseball coach mentioned earlier who identifies gaps in the baseball team's skill set, a team leader in health care must diagnose those gaps, ascertain the potential impact of those gaps on the team's performance, and develop a plan to enhance skills of team members and fill skill gaps.

What Is a Skill Gap?

A skill gap is the difference, or gap, between the skills currently held by an individual or team and the skills needed to meet a future goal. Individuals may note a skill gap between the skills they need to advance in their positions and the skills that they currently possess. Teams may note a skill gap when considering the cumulative skills of the team and the necessary skills for them to succeed with their mission. Regardless of the level of skill gap (individual or team), the gap in skills will likely inhibit success. It is essential to diagnose these gaps promptly and to develop a plan for filling the gap.

Diagnosis of Skill Gaps

A skill gap analysis will be helpful to any team's future success and planning. To perform a skill gap analysis, the steps in performing the analysis for any team are:

1. First, the team should identify all of the skills that will be required in performing the work of the team. Skills that matter will depend on the work of the team. So, for instance, in a team that will rely heavily on technology to complete their work, technological savvy might be a skill that is listed. For teams that must negotiate with a variety of stakeholders to be successful, negotiation, collaboration, and conflict resolution may be skills that would be included at this stage.

TABLE 3.2
Skill Gap Analysis

SKILLS REQUIRED TO MEET TEAM MISSION	LEVEL OF SKILL REQUIRED IN TEAM	DENSITY OF SKILL REQUIRED IN TEAM	SKILL PRESENT IN TEAM (LIST BY NAME AND LEVEL OF SKILL)	SKILL GAP IDENTIFIED

2. Next, for each skill, the team will want to ascertain the required level of that skill, and the team's perception of how pervasive this skill should be within the team. Determining the required level of skill as well as how pervasive the skill must be across team members will allow team leaders to make decisions about how to plan for enhancing that skill in the team. Depending on the identified levels needed for skills, enhancements can range from development of the skill in current team members, to addition of team members with those skills, to adding consultants to the team.

3. Compare the skills needed to meet the team's mission with the team profile that has been developed using the tools provided in Chapter 2 and earlier in this chapter. The team may want to develop a graphic illustration of the identified gaps and the level of need like the one found in Table 3.2.

A simple way for teams to graphically highlight skill gaps is to use color; red indicating highly pervasive or urgent gaps, yellow indicating moderate gaps that may require some development within the team, and green indicating that there is no gap in team skills.

Planning to Enhance Skills and Fill Skill Gaps

Once a team has identified skill gaps, planning to fill those gaps in the most appropriate way for the team, their mission, and their organization should be undertaken. The team has several possible choices for filling the gaps, including developing or increasing expertise within team members, adding team members with expertise in the areas of identified gaps, or adding consultants external to the team to bring these skills to the work of the team. Decisions about how to approach filling the gaps can be guided by the following questions:

Developing or enhancing expertise in current team members:

■ Do current team members have an interest in the development of this skill?

■ Do current team members have the capacity for the development of this skill (time, energy, funding, etc.)?

■ Will the development of this skill in team members further enhance their current skills? Alternatively, will the development of this skill in team members diminish their ability to use other skills needed by the team?

■ Are resources, including time, funding, and expertise to provide development, available to support the development of this skill in current team members?

Adding team members with expertise in the areas of identified skill gaps:

■ Are potential team members who possess the level of expertise in this skill available? Are they available in the organization? Outside of the organization?

■ Do potential team members who possess the level of expertise in this skill have the time available and interest in serving as a member of the team?

■ How will addition of team members impact current team functioning? Will functioning be enhanced? Will functioning be inhibited?

■ How will new members be integrated into the team?

■ Are there additional benefits realized by adding team members?

Adding consultants external to the team to bring skills needed:

■ Are consultants available who possess the expertise needed for the team's work?

■ What is the cost of these consultants? Can the team or organization support these costs?

■ How will introducing a consultant impact the functioning of the team? Will functioning be enhanced? Will functioning be inhibited?

■ How will consultants be integrated into the team?

■ Who will manage the consultant–consultee relationship?

■ Are there additional benefits realized by adding a consultant who is not a member of the team?

The team can use the form found in Table 3.3 to add its plan to address the gaps that were identified in the skill gap analysis.

TABLE 3.3
Skill Gap Analysis With Plan for Addressing Gaps

SKILLS REQUIRED TO MEET TEAM MISSION	LEVEL OF SKILL REQUIRED IN TEAM	DENSITY OF SKILL REQUIRED IN TEAM	SKILL PRESENT IN TEAM (LIST BY NAME AND LEVEL OF SKILL)	SKILL GAP IDENTIFIED	PLAN TO ADDRESS SKILL GAP (WITH SUGGESTED NAMES/CONTACT INFORMATION)
					Develop in team Add team members _____ _____ Consultant _____
					Develop in team Add team members _____ _____ Consultant _____
					Develop in team Add team members _____ _____ Consultant _____
					Develop in team Add team members _____ _____ Consultant _____
					Develop in team Add team members _____ _____ Consultant _____

GAP ANALYSIS EXEMPLAR

The method of gap analysis and planning to enhance skills and fill skill gaps described here was used successfully in a team of stakeholders planning for the development of legislation to support a new state-level nursing workforce center. The team leader was then able to plan a variety of ways to fill the gap. Consider the following case exemplar:

> After studying the impending nursing shortage in a rural state, leaders in nursing and health care appointed to a nursing shortage study commission by the governor developed a number of individual recommendations for strategies to be undertaken to address potential shortages. These ranged from strategies for increasing the pipeline of potential nursing students, to increasing enrollment in nursing programs statewide, to increasing scholarship and loan support, to enhancing the nursing faculty pool through support of graduate education and tax credits for nursing faculty, to addressing the care environment to enhance retention of nurses, to strategies to entice nurses who have left the state to return. In addition, in the study process, the commission noted the challenges of having accurate data about the nursing workforce upon which to make recommendations. Therefore, an additional recommendation was to develop a central data repository for nursing supply-and-demand data. The recommendations were diverse and complex. The main problem with the implementation of the recommendations was that there was no one entity at the state level that had the interest, authority, or funding to make them a reality. Although many stakeholders were "nibbling around the edge" of many of these recommendations at the local level, there still existed a spirit of competition across organizations, as opposed to collaboration for the good of the workforce. The commission decided that developing and empowering a new state agency, in this case a nursing workforce center, would provide the infrastructure to support the development of statewide initiatives to meet the objectives. The commission made a recommendation to the legislature, along with a funding plan; however, no action was taken.
>
> Several stakeholder organizations that were involved in the commission were not willing to allow the work of the commission to be forgotten. After meeting to discuss next

TABLE 3.4
Skill Gap Analysis (With Plan for Addressing Gaps)

SKILLS REQUIRED TO MEET TEAM MISSION	LEVEL OF SKILL REQUIRED IN TEAM	DENSITY OF SKILL REQUIRED IN TEAM	SKILL PRESENT IN TEAM (LIST BY NAME AND LEVEL OF SKILL)	SKILL GAP IDENTIFIED	PLAN TO ADDRESS SKILL GAP (WITH SUGGESTED NAMES/ CONTACT INFORMATION)
Knowledge of existing data and data analysis techniques	Expert	At least one member must be an expert for analysis and presentation	Team leader expert		**Develop in team** Data 101 for all team members
	Moderate	All team members must understand data	Half of team expresses need for further skill to understand complex data	YES	**Add team members** ____ ____ ____ **Consultant**
Ability to build consensus with a variety of stakeholders, including nursing higher education, practice (public and private), health care agencies (rural, urban, tertiary care, primary care, etc.), health care advocates (professional organizations, citizen groups), medical specialties with legislative power	Expert	Must have team members with expertise in each area	Have team member from public education	YES Need team member from private nursing education, K–12 education, medical specialties, other professional advocacy groups	**Develop in team**
					Add team members
			Small hospital		**Nurse educator from privately funded school**
			Large hospital		
			Long-term care		**K–12 educator**
			Public health		
			Citizen advocacy		**Medical association, other professional groups**
			Professional advocacy (Nurses Association)		**Consultant** ____ ____ ____

(continued)

TABLE 3.4

Skill Gap Analysis (With Plan for Addressing Gaps) *(continued)*

SKILLS REQUIRED TO MEET TEAM MISSION	LEVEL OF SKILL REQUIRED IN TEAM	DENSITY OF SKILL REQUIRED IN TEAM	SKILL PRESENT IN TEAM (LIST BY NAME AND LEVEL OF SKILL)	SKILL GAP IDENTIFIED	PLAN TO ADDRESS SKILL GAP (WITH SUGGESTED NAMES/ CONTACT INFORMATION)
Public speaking	Expert	At least several members with expertise	All members comfortable, one member designated spokesperson	NO	**Develop in team** **Add team members** Consultant
Financial expertise to analyze costs of startup of new center, funding sources	Expert	At least one to two members must possess expertise	None	YES	**Develop in team** **Add team members** Consultant **Add financial consultant with legislative experience**

Skill/experience needed	Level	Requirement	Current team status	Have it?	Action
Experience with legislative process, including providing education, presenting to legislative committees, writing legislation for introduction, lobbying, building support, negotiation	Expert/moderate	All members must have some level of expertise	One professional lobbyist on team, three other team members with lobbying experience, three team members comfortable with developing educational materials for policy support	YES	**Develop in team** Lobbying 101 for all team members _____ **Add team members** _____ _____ **Consultant** _____ _____

steps, one organization agreed to take the lead on pushing forward legislation for the workforce center, and a member of that organization was designated as the team leader. A variety of organizations volunteered to work toward the introduction and passage of the legislation, believing it was for the good of the state. The group adopted the mission of "successfully introducing, supporting, and passing legislation to lead to the eventual formation of a nursing workforce center to be empowered to address the nursing shortage through data collection, recruitment and retention initiatives." At the first meeting, the group undertook a skills analysis to identify the skills that existed in the group. Next, they identified the skills that would be necessary to meet their mission. Finally, they developed a plan to fill the skill gaps identified in their team. The full gap analysis and plan is found in Table 3.4.

Through use of this simple tool, forethought, and planning, this team was built for success. In the second legislative session after the team began to work together, legislation was unanimously passed to create the nursing workforce center. The center has been in place for over 6 years, and stakeholders on the original team have continued to support the work of the center.

SUMMARY AND NEXT STEPS

In this chapter, we have analyzed how preferences of individual team members related to teaming can be translated by leaders into actions to build the strongest team possible. Multiple methods for analyzing team strengths and skills are available for team leaders to purposefully develop teams that are built for success. In the next chapters, we will analyze strategies and actions for team success as the team begins its work together in nursing and health care environments.

QUESTIONS FOR THOUGHT

1. Develop a plan for your team to analyze talents and skills. Consider a mix of self-analysis, observational techniques, and formal skills assessment in your plan.
2. Conduct a mock interview for a potential team member. Plan your interview questions to assess individual skills and talents.
3. Devise a plan to analyze and fill skill gaps in your team. What skills are needed? What skills are missing? How will you enhance the skills of your team to fill the identified gaps?

FOUR

Team Strategies for Success in Nursing and Health Care Environments

There ain't no rules here. We're trying to accomplish something.
—Thomas Edison

LEARNING OBJECTIVES

1. Discuss the impact of the work environment on a team, including the concepts of professionalism and relational coordination.
2. Analyze internal team structures and processes that can impact team success.
3. Devise a team charter, mission, vision, goals, and ground rules.
4. Identify ways to deal with team conflict.
5. Apply measures of transparency to teamwork.
6. Understand the normal trajectory of team development.

Critical to the success of the work of a team is the environment in which the team functions. Health care and nursing leaders, as well as teams and their leaders can create an environment for success. A balance of external supports and internal structures can facilitate a team's work and the outcomes it can produce. The impact of professionalism and relational coordination as external environmental factors impacting the work of a team cannot be underestimated. Likewise, internal team structures, such as a team charter, mission and vision, goals, ground rules, methods to handle conflict, and transparency can be essential to the accomplishment of the team's goals. Finally, an understanding of the normal trajectory of team development can assist a team in understanding the natural course of a team's growth.

THE IMPACT OF PROFESSIONALISM

An environment of professionalism is a key component of success in any organization. But an environment of professionalism requires dedication to the tenets of professionalism by everyone in the organization. It should be no surprise that the components of professionalism will also lead to team success. But, what are these components, and how does a team leader facilitate a professional environment? Honesty and integrity, reliability and responsibility, respect for others, compassion and empathy, dedication to self-improvement, self-awareness and knowledge of one's own limits, communication and collaboration, and advocacy are some of the essential components of professionalism to be considered by every team.

Honesty and Integrity

Team members must have consistent regard for the highest standards in their work. Work should not ever be considered "good enough," but rather team members should always strive for excellence. This involves meeting commitments, dedication to the work of the team, and giving 110% at all times. Honesty and integrity also require a refusal to ever violate one's personal and professional codes of ethics. Team leaders and members should dedicate themselves to the highest ethical standards in their work. They also should be forthright in their interactions with each other, with peers, with other professionals, and with patients and families. Finally, team leaders and members need to be aware of any conflict of interest or situations that may result in personal gain at the expense of others. When a conflict of interest arises, or even if the appearance of a conflict of interest is possible, team members should disclose the conflict, and frank discussion about the ramifications of the conflict should be undertaken and actions for the team to avoid conflict of interest should occur. Conflicts of interest can occur in a variety of different ways, including advocating for positions based on the potential for personal gain, making decisions that will result in financial gains for themselves or their family or close friends, or evaluating products or services with bias due to outside relationships. Remember, even the appearance of a conflict of interest should be disclosed to the team, allowing the team to decide how to deal with potential conflicts. All actions of the team should be approached in a spirit of striving for honesty and integrity.

Reliability and Responsibility

Teams must be reliable in their work, and must commit to the goals and work of the team. Team members must commit to being accountable to the team and for their actions. Accountability extends to the team, but beyond the team to every stakeholder in the team's work. These stakeholders may include patients, peers, employers, and the profession. Teams must be willing to accept responsibility for the successes and failures of the team. Teams must be willing to accept responsibility for errors, and committed to correcting those errors. Finally, team members must be committed to doing their best possible work, every time they work as a team.

A lack of reliability and responsibility can unravel the bonds of a team quicker than any other action. When team members cannot keep up their end of the work of the team, team members can become resentful and angry. The responsible team leader will deal with unreliable team members quickly, exploring the reasons for the unreliable behavior with the team member, and developing possible remedies that will allow the team to stay intact. However, the team leader may also want to consider the possibility that the team will function more effectively without the unreliable team member, and should be prepared to explore this possibility with the team members as well. Team leaders must continuously consider what is "best for the team," and take actions to assure the team's most effective functioning.

Respect for Others

Humanism, or respect for others, is central to the concept of professionalism. Respect extends to all spheres of the team's contact, whether it is contact with other team members, team leaders, sponsors or mentors, other peers and professionals, patients, families, or the community at large. In a professional environment, everyone is treated with regard for individual worth and dignity, with respect for the strengths each member brings to the work of the team. In an environment of respect, confidentiality is observed, but more important, the work of the team is treated with respect, regardless of whether individual team members agree completely with all plans or actions of the team.

An awareness of the various influences on team member actions, organizational choices, and a respect for differences is integral to team success. These influences may include personal, cultural, political, and emotional factors, and should be respected and embraced in a professional environment. The team leader should actively seek out awareness of the influences that may impact a team member's actions. For instance, consider the team that is working together on developing the portfolio required for a hospital's Magnet designation application, and is having a difficult time carving out time during the work week to complete the work. A team member suggests that perhaps they could meet on Friday evenings to work, given that no one on the team needs to work on Saturday, so they could work long into the evening. What personal, cultural, religious, or other considerations should the team leader consider when acting in a respectful, professional manner? Perhaps one team member has a teen who is a star football player, and they play games on Friday evening. Perhaps one team member is Jewish, and their Sabbath begins on Friday at sundown, after which no work can occur. Selecting Friday evenings for work of the team may systematically discriminate against these team members, who have two choices—to ignore their personal, cultural, or religious commitments and work with the team, or to miss the team meetings, potentially being seen by other team members as unreliable. The respectful team leader considers these differences when making decisions that will affect team members—embracing diversity in the team, while respecting team members' individual differences.

Compassion and Empathy

In an environment of professionalism, team members are attentive to diversity within the team, and to the influences on the behavior of individuals. Team members respond in humane ways, trying to relieve discomfort of members and stakeholders, or to quell anxieties that may occur during the work of the team. Open discussion of diversity and of personal limitations on time and effort can be facilitated by the team member and can help the team's eventual success.

Self-Improvement

Team members and leaders in a professional environment are committed to lifelong learning. This commitment includes aspirations toward excellence in all that team members strive to accomplish. Team members should be supported in training related to the core function of the team. Equally as important though is education related to team development, team functioning, and team evaluation.

Self-evaluation and acceptance of critique and feedback from others is essential to begin the path toward self-improvement. Development of a team improvement plan will be informed by individual self-evaluation and individual plans for improvement.

Self-Awareness and Knowledge of Limits

Self-awareness in a professional environment requires insight into how one's behavior impacts others in the team. Closely linked to an understanding of one's behaviors is an understanding of the scope of practice of all members of the team, and professional boundaries that may be important to the work of the team. This is especially important in interprofessional teams, where the scope of practice of individuals may vary widely, and may impact the actions that each team member is able to pursue, based on education, certification, or licensure.

Recognition of the need for guidance or supervision when confronted by new or complex responsibilities is also key to an environment of professionalism. Team members must learn to recognize their limits, and to seek out expertise inside or outside of the team to enhance their understanding and knowledge in a particular area. Team leaders should serve as role models for seeking guidance when needed. Guidance may be sought within the team, or outside of the team depending on the nature of the problem. For instance, new team leaders may seek guidance from members of the team who have functioned in leadership roles in the past, especially when dealing with issues that are outside of the team, for instance, how to influence stakeholders. When dealing with an internal team issue, for example, an unreliable team member, team leaders may want to seek assistance from outside of the team from other team leaders. In this case, seeking assistance within the team may be difficult, as team members' responses may be influenced by team dynamics.

Advocacy

In a professional environment, devotion to the welfare of others should be obvious. Teams should be dedicated to taking action to assure the welfare of others, including team members, stakeholders, the organization, and the profession. The key to advocacy in a professional environment is sharing of knowledge, speaking up on behalf of others, and serving as a catalyst for change. Team leaders can role model this behavior within the team, pointing out team members' talents and contributions.

Outside of the team, team leaders can advocate for positions that support the team's goals with key sponsors and stakeholders.

Communication and Collaboration

Probably the most important tenet of a professional environment for team success is the ability to communicate and a dedication to collaborate to meet the goals of the team. Effective communication extends to team members and peers, other professionals and all stakeholders in the team's work. Specific to team communication, team members in a professional environment understand that team success begins with the clear communication of their needs, and the needs of their stakeholders. They also understand the need to work collaboratively and cooperatively in a proactive manner to meet those needs.

OPERATIONALIZING A PROFESSIONAL ENVIRONMENT FOR TEAM SUCCESS

Sometimes, teams need a road map to operationalize the components of professionalism within a team. Team leaders can facilitate a professionalism inventory like the one in Table 4.1 at any time during the team's development. At the beginning of a team's work together, a professionalism inventory can help to set the stage for a healthy team environment. At later stages of a team's development, the same inventory can help team members step back and analyze their work together, the influences on that work, and to develop a plan for future success.

After taking some time to individually take inventory of personal aspects of professionalism, team members can begin to thoughtfully plan for how to improve the professional environment for their work. Team members can evaluate where they excel, and can also identify ways they can improve the professional environment. Some strategies for improvement will be suggested later in this chapter in the development of a team charter, mission, vision, goals, and ground rules. Any strategies, however, will require commitment, support, and leadership.

Commitment

Team members should make a realistic plan to impact the professional environment in which they work and commit to that plan. The plan should include strategies for improving the professional environment, and could be as simple as "we will commit to respecting

TABLE 4.1
Professionalism Inventory

WHEN WAS THE LAST TIME YOU	WHEN WERE YOU LAST
Personally or as a team sought out an education experience to improve your knowledge?	Proactive about your needs or the needs of your peers, your team, your unit, your patients or their families?
Read your professional Code of Ethics?	Aware of the influence of your culture, your education, your beliefs on your interactions with others in the team?
Participated in the work of an outside professional organization to expand your knowledge?	Accountable to your team?
Communicated your knowledge to others in any format (team meeting, presentation, publication)?	Forthright in your interactions with others?
Consciously evaluated your needs and communicated them to others?	Aware of a need to seek outside assistance when faced with responsibilities outside of your knowledge limits?
Accepted or provided thoughtful feedback from others?	A catalyst for change?
Considered how your behavior affects others in the team?	Cognizant and respectful of professional boundaries?
Were attentive to the anxiety of others on the team?	A collaborator?

other's time by being on time for meetings." Strategies should be lived each and every day of the team's work together. Frank discussions about gaps in professionalism will lead to improvements in the professional environment.

Support

Once a commitment to a professional environment has been made, teams should support each other in their commitment. Mechanisms for supporting the plan for a professional environment should be sought. For the simple commitment to be on time for meetings, one mechanism for support might be the use of an electronic calendar entry for all team members along with a reminder alarm 15 minutes before the meeting. Supports need not be elaborate, but can be creatively deployed to facilitate a professional environment.

Leadership

In the case of development and support of a professional environment, all team members must serve as leaders. Professionalism depends on each individual taking responsibility for one's own behavior, and for facilitating the environment of professionalism in the group. In 2000, Ramona Sharpnak, a mentor to many women leaders in influential companies across the country, said in an interview in *Fast Company* magazine, *"to be a leader, don't worry so much about what you need to know. Instead, figure out who you need to be"* (Dahl, 2000). These words are particularly important when considering an environment of professionalism—each person on the team must lead by his or her professional actions and attitudes.

RELATIONAL COORDINATION

Relational coordination is a term that has been defined by Gittell (2002) in Havens, Vasey, Gittell, and Lin (2010) as a "mutually reinforcing process of interaction between communication and relationships carried out for the purpose of task integration" (p. 18). Simply put, coordination of activities in a team relies not only on communication, but also on relationships among team members. The dimensions of relational coordination as delineated by Havens and colleagues (2010) can easily be applied to the work of teams. Teams must communicate about their work frequently, in a timely manner, accurately depicting their work and progress, and in a problem-solving, rather than a blaming manner. Key to relational coordination is that these communication techniques are coupled with shared goals, shared knowledge, and a mutual respect for the work of other team members. Havens and colleagues (2010) and others (Bacon et al., 2009; Bae, Mark, & Fried, 2010; Gittell et al., 2000; Gittell, Godfrey, & Thistlewaite, 2012) have linked through their research the impact of relational coordination on patient care quality outcomes, including overall quality of care, decreased adverse events, and patient satisfaction with care. In a recent publication, Gittell et al. (2012) documented the impact of interprofessional collaborative practice and relational coordination on improved health care outcomes.

> The documentation of these patient care outcomes as a result of relational coordination support the need for attention to management of communication and relationships within the health care team.

OPERATIONALIZING RELATIONAL COORDINATION IN TEAMS

Two main sets of processes are thought to result in relational coordination—communication and relationships (including shared goals, shared knowledge, and mutual respect). What can team leaders do to facilitate these processes and thus assure more positive outcomes for the team?

Communication: If we examine the main components of communication in the model found in Figure 4.1, we can see that frequent, timely, and accurate communication that is focused on problem solving is the key to relational coordination. Leaders and team members can use techniques from the simple to complex to facilitate this type of communication. Setting up regular meetings (such as the "Scrum" process described in Chapter 6) and using electronic forms of communication such as e-mail, social media, or shared electronic sites are relatively simple. Using technology to share data and work products could range from simple e-mails to team members, to using more sophisticated sharing sites such as Microsoft's SharePoint (www.sharepoint.microsoft.com/en-us/Pages/default.aspx), DropBox™ (www.dropbox.com/teams), and others. These "cloud"-based technologies allow multiple team members to communicate across time-and-distance barriers or

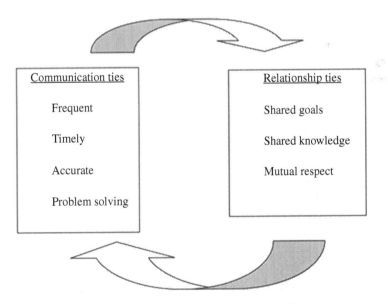

FIGURE 4.1 Dimensions of relational coordination.

Source: Reprinted from Havens et al. (2010), with permission from Blackwell Publishing Ltd.

within the same organization. Basically, communications, papers, working products, or virtually any file application can be saved to these systems and accessed by any member of the team, no matter where he or she is in the world. Products can be saved over unlimited time, allowing for a repository of the team's work. New team members can get quickly up to speed by reviewing documents in the cloud system. Sharing of best practices is facilitated across the team or across an organization. Of course, the use of any technology within an organization must be approved by organizational information technology leaders, and must be compatible with systems already existing within the organization.

Below is a screenshot of a typical Dropbox™ site set up to share documents among a research team. All team members have access, and once they are invited by the team leader to download Dropbox™, they are provided with password-protected access to all items saved on the site regardless of where they are in the world. Documents are saved by simply selecting Dropbox™ as the site to save to, just like saving any other document, adding simplicity to the communication process (Figure 4.2).

A recent white paper on the use of Microsoft SharePoint, another cloud-based sharing site, reported an examination of three Fortune 500 companies and the outcomes of their teams realized through implementation (Mainstay Partners, 2011). Findings included a broader sense of collaboration across teams, the ability to give all team members a voice, and a sense of empowerment of all team members when Microsoft SharePoint was used in a variety of different ways. Words

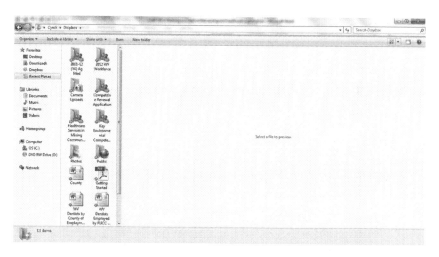

FIGURE 4.2 Sample Dropbox™ site for team document sharing.

that companies used to describe the changes in their teams included "bonds," "better communication," and "higher levels of trust" (p. 8). Team leaders can use these innovations in technology to enhance communication in their teams.

Relationships

In the relational coordination model just presented, shared goals, shared trust, and mutual respect are key components of relationships. We also know from our examination of teams in Chapter 1 that these are key characteristics of teams. How does the team leader facilitate shared goals, shared trust, and mutual respect? Internal team structures, such as a team charter, mission and vision, goals, ground rules, methods to handle conflict, and transparency can be essential to the accomplishment of the team's goals of relationship building.

TEAM CHARTER

Ideally developed at the beginning of a team's work together, multiple reasons exist for preparing a team charter. One is to document the team's purpose and define roles, responsibilities, and rules of operation. The team charter also establishes procedures for the team and the organization on communication, reporting, and decision-making processes. The team charter may delineate deliverables to be created by the team. The team charter empowers the team by including team responsibility and authority (Mikes, 2010). Figure 4.3 provides a template that a team might use to create its charter (www.acquisitions. gov). Figure 4.4 is a sample team charter developed by a nursing team.

Completing the team charter early can facilitate shared goals, shared knowledge of each member's skills and talents, and mutual trust among team members. Consider the sample team charter in Figure 4.4 developed by a team charged with developing a Professional Practice Model to enhance patient care quality and improve provider satisfaction in a mid-size hospital. At their first meeting, a retreat to kick off their work, this team undertook the development of a team charter. As you review this team charter, consider what we have learned in previous chapters about selection of team members for varied expertise, organizational considerations when implementing team processes, and the importance of shared goals. It becomes obvious when reviewing this charter that this team has done its homework and is ready to begin its work together in an effective way.

TEAM CHARTER

The charter includes the following sections:

1. Purpose

(Describe the purpose for forming the team and the anticipated outcomes.)

2. Background

(Summarize the program or project the team is supporting, state how the team fits within the organizational structure, identify who are the users or intended recipients of the program or project including external stakeholders.)

3. Scope

(State the scope, mission, and objectives for the team. This is similar to preparing a mission or need statement. Define the high-level goals the team must accomplish.)

4. Team composition

(Who is a part of the team? Identify the functional areas and organizational components represented, the number of members from each, state who are core [essential] members versus support or advisory members, and the anticipated time/resource and commitments involved over the anticipated duration of the team.)

5. Membership roles

(Identify roles and responsibilities of each team member. List member name, organization, contact information, including telephone and e-mail address, and team role if designated already. Also identify specific functional level of expertise associated with each member.)

6. Team empowerment

(Define existing authority of the team and additional authority needed to fully perform as envisioned by the team objectives.)

7. Team operations

(Describe team operational plans. This includes, for example, such activities as the team's decision-making processes, how changes in membership occur should the need arise, plans to establish "ground" or operating rules, relationships with other organizational teams, team support, etc.)

8. Team performance assessment

(Document key areas of performance needed for team success along with means of measuring progress.)

9. Activity milestones and schedules

(Include major activities and milestones forecasted along with associated time frames and schedule.)

10. Signature page

(Each team member signs, agreeing to the contents and being held mutually accountable for adherence.)

11. Approval

(Individuals authorized to approve the team charter sign with their approval.)

FIGURE 4.3 Template for team charter.

Source: Adapted from *Generic Team Charter Template*, Retrieved from www.acquisitions.gov

TEAM CHARTER FOR ST. THOMAS HOSPITAL PROFESSIONAL PRACTICE MODEL DEVELOPMENT TEAM

Purpose

St. Thomas Hospital has undertaken a process to develop a Professional Practice Model to guide the work of our patient care providers, teams, and departments. We expect that the results of implementing a Professional Practice Model will be improved quality of care for those we serve and enhanced satisfaction of the providers in our system. Our mission to be the provider of choice because of the quality of care we provide in our region will be supported by the implementation of the Professional Practice Model. A team of stakeholders from our patient care departments has been formed to develop the Professional Practice Model for our organization, considering the best evidence and the best fit for our organization.

Background

The Professional Practice Model team will support the development of the Professional Practice Model for the organization. The team reports directly to the vice president for Patient Care Services. The Professional Practice Model will impact all professional care providers in the organization, and the work of those providers has the potential to impact all patients and families we serve.

Scope

The team's mission is to develop a Professional Practice Model that is a fit for the organization. The team's objectives are to:

1. Review the literature for Professional Practice Models used in similar health care organizations, their components, and documented outcomes resulting from their implementation.
2. Benchmark with similar health care organizations for Professional Practice Model implementation, successes, and barriers.
3. Assess our staff's wants and needs related to a Professional Practice Model.
4. Compare the components of identified Professional Practice Models to the culture and structure of our organization.
5. Evaluate the efficacy of each model in our organization.
6. Propose the implementation of the model, or a hybrid of several models that has been identified as the best fit for our organization.
7. Develop a system-wide plan for implementation of the model.
8. Develop outcome measures to evaluate the model's impact on patient care and provider satisfaction.

Team Composition

The team is composed of one representative from each nursing Council (Quality, Education, Evidence-Based Practice, and Retention), and one representative of each other patient care area (Pharmacy, Radiology, Patient Care Support Services, Laboratory Services). The VP for Patient Care Services, director of Quality, and the director of Human Resources are advisory members of the committee. Anticipated time and resource commitments include 1-hour weekly meetings for the next 6 months, a kickoff retreat of 1 day, and information and data resources of the Councils and Departments.

FIGURE 4.4 Sample team charter.

Membership Roles

TEAM MEMBER NAME	DEPARTMENT	CONTACT INFORMATION	TEAM ROLE	FUNCTIONAL EXPERTISE
Joe	Quality Council		Chairperson	Public speaking, quality measures, relationship building
Jane	Education Council		TBA	Curriculum development, learner evaluation
Clara	Evidence-Based Practice Council		TBA	Review of literature, analysis and synthesis of best practices, presentation development
Susan	Retention Council		TBA	System-based decision making, strategic planning, provider satisfaction measurement
David	Pharmacy		Vice Chairperson	Systems and process development, relationship building, coalition development
John	Radiology		TBA	External stakeholder relationships
Eric	Patient Support Services			Big-picture view of organization
Aaron	Laboratory			Complex system evaluation, public speaking
Pat	VP Patient Care Services		Advisory	Access to resources, liaison to higher levels of administration
Ron	Director of Quality		Advisory	Quality measurement and evaluation
Barb	Director of Human Resources		Advisory	Best practices for provider satisfaction, Staff assessment

FIGURE 4.4 *(continued)*

Team Empowerment

The team exists under the authority of the vice president for Patient Care Services, who is charged with assuring delivery of the best possible care to those we serve. The team has been given full authority to initiate all processes needed to achieve its objectives. Advisory members of the team will assist the team in developing the best possible model for implementation, implementation processes, and resources necessary to accomplish the goals.

Team Operations

The team will operate using consensus for decision making. Expertise of each team member will be utilized and respected by the team. If team members leave the organization or the team, the team will select replacement members from the appropriate organizational entity to assure full representation of all patient care areas on the team. As much as possible, the team will select members who enhance the skills and talents of the team. The team will develop ground rules for team functioning within the first month of its existence. The team will work across the organization, primarily through the liaison roles of its members to each of their respective patient care areas. Team staff support will be provided by the Administrative Associate for Patient Care Services.

Team Performance Assessment

Key to the team's success will be high-level performance in the area of communication, mutual respect, and shared goals. The team will agree to systems that will allow attainment of their goals. Progress toward goals will be assessed each week at the team meeting, and overall progress toward goal completion will be assessed monthly.

Activity Milestones and Schedules
(Phase 1: Literature review, benchmarking, staff survey)

ACTIVITIES	TIME FRAME	RESPONSIBLE TEAM MEMBERS
Review of literature initiated.	Month 1	Clara, Joe, Ron
Review of literature completed.	Month 2	Clara, Joe, Ron
Benchmark survey developed.	Month 1	John, Eric, Aaron
Benchmark survey with 15 peer institutions completed and analyzed.	Month 2	John, Eric, Aaron
Staff survey developed.	Month 1	Susan, David, Jane
Staff survey completed and analyzed.	Month 2	Susan, David, Jane

Signatures of Team Members

_____   _____
_____   _____
_____   _____
_____   _____

Approval

_____   _____
VP for Patient Care Services   CEO

FIGURE 4.4 *(continued)*

TEAM MISSION AND VISION

Closely related to some of the elements of the team charter, and informing the work of the team, are the team's mission and vision. An organization may have a broad mission and vision, and the team's mission and vision, although related to that of the organization, will be much more specific to the team's purpose, as is included in the team charter. Mission and vision statements serve specific purposes within a team, including:

- Describing the overall purpose of the team: what the team does, who they do it for, and how and why they do it.
- Setting the boundaries of the team's activities.
- Forming the starting point in developing a vision.

A mission review gets a team back to basics. The essential activity of determining who a team serves can be a wake-up call for teams that have started to skew their activities to meet the needs of other stakeholders (such as their funders), and not their sponsors. The team whose charter is included in this chapter developed the mission statement below:

> Our mission is to develop a professional practice model based on best evidence that is designed to guide patient and family care at St. Thomas Hospital, improve the quality of patient care and satisfaction of providers in our system.

This mission fulfills the requirements of a team mission statement. The team has identified what the team does (*develop a professional practice model to guide patient and family care*), who they do it for (*St. Thomas Hospital*), and how (*based on best evidence*) and why they do it (*improve the quality of patient care and the satisfaction of providers in our system*). The team can use this mission statement to determine when it is moving outside of its scope, for instance, if the team begins to focus more on organizational structures than professional practice models, revisiting their mission could help them refocus on their core purpose for existing.

The team vision should describe an ideal future for the team or the result of the team's work. It is the "big picture" that is so often referred to in an organization. Bigger than a mission, the vision answers the question, what impact do we want to have on the greater organization? Visions give a team or an organization a common, coherent strategic direction. Some say that a vision conveys a larger sense of purpose, so that team members see themselves as "building a home" rather than "laying bricks." Finally, a vision has the "gulp" factor—when it dawns on team members what it will take to achieve the goal and the level of commitment to the goal, there should be an almost audible gulp (Collins & Porras, 1996, p. 75).

The team whose charter is set in the preceding text adopted the following vision statement for its work:

> St. Thomas Hospital will become the premier provider of quality health care in the state through the use of a professional practice model.

In evaluating this vision statement, one needs consider whether it includes the qualities of a true vision statement. It is "big picture," unites a team in a common purpose, relates back to the organization, and should produce an audible gulp—the work of the team can potentially impact the entire organization and the health of the state!

TEAM GROUND RULES

To effectively work together to fulfill the mission of the team, and to realize the vision established by the team, ground rules should be considered for the team's work. Team ground rules are a set of agreed-upon rules that reflect how a team agrees to work together. Ground rules are an essential component of team operation. Setting ground rules from the beginning of a team's work together will facilitate a shared understanding of how the team operates, increasing trust from the outset. Going back and setting up rules once a team has encountered a problem will hinder the team's effectiveness. Taking the time to set ground rules early in a team's work together will pay off in the long term.

Ground rules form a safe environment for team functioning. Team ground rules can establish norms that describe how the team will work together with each other to meet their goals. Here are some steps that teams might use to establish ground rules:

1. Set aside time at the first team meeting to discuss ground rules. Make sure everyone understands what a ground rule is. Leaders might want to have a list of common ground rules available to get the discussion started. For instance, some teams automatically accept "We will start our meetings on time, and adjourn on time"

as a basic ground rule. Other teams agree that all team meetings will have a published agenda, allowing all team members to understand the goals of the meeting as they relate to the work of the team. Some teams like to have ground rules that allow the team to assign roles for each meeting, helping them work effectively together. So, a ground rule might be written that says "at each meeting, we will assign a recorder, a time keeper, and a ground rules monitor." Although the team should collectively develop and agree to the ground rules, sometimes a leader can get the process started by offering a commonly agreed-upon goal to begin the discussion.

2. Be sure that rules reflect what is important to team members. What do they value? A team that values participation by all members might include a rule that says "We will all promise to be active participants in every meeting, and we will encourage the participation of all through our actions." A team that wants to encourage mutual respect might adopt a ground rule that says "Ranks are left at the door," which allows all team members to participate on equal footing within the team. Teams who value staying on track during meetings may develop a ground rule that says "when we get off topic, or are confronted with an issue we cannot deal with at this time, we will place it in a 'parking lot' and will revisit it later in our work."

3. The team should also consider what is not acceptable to the team. A team might decide that talking badly outside of the team about the team's work is absolutely unacceptable. So, a ground rule for that team might be "We agree that our decisions are made by consensus, and we will not speak badly of the work of the team once we leave the room." A team focused on safety in a direct patient care environment might agree to a common ground rule that says "Anyone on the team can call a timeout at any time to assure safe patient care."

4. Although open debate is essential for a team's work, conflict can undermine the attainment of a team's goals. Ground rules about addressing conflict in the team are essential. What conflict resolution model will you use? What do teams value in resolving conflict? At a minimum, teams will want to set a ground rule related to respecting one another despite conflict. Other ground rules such as "We will speak from our hearts, and listen attentively to one another" may be helpful. Models such as the Interest-Based Relational (IBR) Approach (Slaikeu, 1996) to conflict resolution might be adopted in ground rules. This model may result in ground rules that support the importance

of relationships, keeping people and problems separate, paying attention to the positions that are being presented, active listening, establishing the facts and objectives, and exploring options together.

5. Another important step in the ground rules process is deciding how the rules will be enforced. Teams will want to decide on a process for maintaining mutual respect while pointing out violations. Some teams decide on a system that will allow anyone on the team to point out a breach in ground rules. One team uses small "stop signs" that can be held up by anyone who believes that a ground rule has been breached—stopping the activity of the team until the team recognizes and corrects actions that breach ground rules. This team found that the stop signs were used more frequently in the beginning of their work, and less frequently as the team matured. Regardless of the process decided upon by the team, pointing out violations of ground rules needs to be timely and direct.

6. Once ground rules have been developed, all team members need to agree to the rules. So, although a process of brainstorming and discussion might result in a list of rules, the most important step is agreement and buy-in.

7. Once ground rules have been agreed upon, decide how the ground rules will be kept front and center for the team. Some teams begin every meeting by reviewing the ground rules and making sure everyone is still in agreement with the rules. New rules may be adopted as the team matures. Other teams post their ground rules in their meeting rooms. Still others have ground rules copied onto every agenda for team meetings. Regardless of the method chosen by the team, ground rules should be reviewed and affirmed frequently by the team.

8. One last step involves orientation of new team members to the ground rules. The team should decide in advance how it will introduce new team members to the ground rules, and how it will include the values of new team members in its review and revision of ground rules for the team.

TEAM TRANSPARENCY

Team transparency is a term that has been commonly defined as an understanding of the work of other members of the team. Joint projects in teams based on voluntary contributions of effort by all team members can be vulnerable to "free-riding." In formulating incentives, a team leader may try to influence its members' efforts by designing the structure of contributions. In particular, the team leader may be able to determine how much the members know about each other's efforts. This type of knowledge can be facilitated by the work environment of the team, such as an open space work environment or regular reporting of team members' actual performance and products to the team (Bag & Pepito, 2012). Transparency in efforts within a team may help to reduce unreliability in team members and foster cooperation. Evidence exists that supports this kind of transparency as a key determinant of productive efficiency in teams in a variety of industries (Falk & Ichino, 2006; Teasley, Covi, Krishnan, & Olsonino, 2002). When team members' efforts are observable during a team's work together (i.e., in a transparent environment), team members tend to work in complementary fashion, increasing their output. If team members are not aware of the efforts of others, team members tend to work in a more sustainable fashion, only working hard enough to sustain output. In operationalizing a transparent environment within the team, the team leader influences the work of each member of the team and incentivizes higher output among team members.

TEAM DEVELOPMENT TRAJECTORY

Even if a team has developed a professional environment, a team charter, goals, mission, vision, and has set up systems to facilitate transparency and complementary work, a team will go through predictable stages in its growth and development. Tuckman (1965) has described these states as *forming, storming, norming, and performing*. The stages have been further illustrated with directional arrows documenting the normal progression of development in Figure 4.5.

Tuckman developed this model in the mid-1960s. In Tuckman's model of team development, the stage of *norming* is typically the first stage of development that the team experiences. In the *norming* stage, teams are beginning to work together, learning about each other and the mission of the team. During the *norming* stage of the team's development, team members set up their team charter, develop their mission and vision, and develop their operating ground rules. During this stage, the team heavily depends on the team leader for direction. Team leaders set the stage for teamwork through developing a professional environment and role modeling the behavior expected of team members. As mentioned in our discussion of team ground rules, team leaders may need to provide direction to teams during the norming

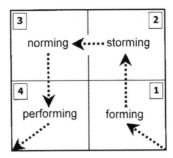

FIGURE 4.5 Tuckman's team development model.
Source: From Tuckman (1965).

stage through providing samples, templates, and examples from other teams' work. The team leader will spend a lot of time providing education about basic team functions such as mission development. The team leader should expect a lot of questions, and need for support. Gaining clarity around the team's purpose is a key component of this stage of development. Leaders might experience some pushback or questioning by team members as they get to know the team leader. The leader will need to be directive with team members during this stage of development as team roles and responsibilities are established.

The next stage, termed *storming* by Tuckman, is, as the name suggests, a turbulent time in the team's development. Team members are trying to establish themselves within the team and with the leader, and may vie for attention and position. Although the purpose of the team established during the forming phase may become clearer, plenty of uncertainties continue. How decisions will actually be made, focus maintained, and ground rules honored is still unclear to team members, and will evolve during this stage. Decision making is difficult for team members, as they are feeling the pressure of getting to know one another, and attempting to put their strengths to best use in the team. There may be power struggles that ensue during this process, with team members sometimes establishing relationships with smaller groups within the team (usually those most like themselves), allowing a clique-like structure to ensue. The team leader must coach the team during this phase of development in order to keep the team focused on the goals they have set, as opposed to focused on emotions and relationships. The team leaders should role model compromise and embrace diversity among group members, coaching all team members to work from their strengths. This is an excellent opportunity to perform some of the assessments of individual team member strengths and preferences, and share these with the group to enable them to get to know each other more quickly and with more precision than just observation. The team leader can help the team to use this information to formulate the team development plan as discussed in Chapters 2 and 3.

The third stage of development according to Tuckman is *norming*. During this stage, a team has settled into its roles, understands its responsibilities, and begins to work together toward meeting its goals. Big decisions are made by the team, and because trust has increased between and among team members, smaller decisions may be delegated to smaller groups, task forces, or even to an individual team member with strengths in the topic. The team has "clicked" and has developed smooth processes for working together, embracing the styles and strengths of everyone involved. At this point in the leadership of the team, the leader becomes a facilitator, helping to enable the team's work through setting processes or resources in place for team success. Because unity is high at this point in development, the team leader may plan fun or social events for the team, and may explore some additional team-building exercises for the team to continue its development. The team leader can also establish times to celebrate and recognize accomplishments of team members, increasing transparency of the work of the team, and facilitating the continued complementary functioning of team members. Finally, the team leader may begin to discuss with the team a plan for continued evaluation of its efforts as a team, so as to continue the team's development. Receptivity to evaluation will be high during the norming stage of team development.

The final stage of team development in Tuckman's original model is *performing*. This is the most effective stage of team development in terms of meeting team goals. Teams understand very clearly what they are doing, why they are doing it, and the benefit of their work in the larger organization. The team functions independently, and needs little more than oversight and delegation from the leader. The team is autonomous in all its functions, including working toward its goals, but also in dealing with disagreement and conflict, as well as setting up processes and systems to achieve their goal. The team leader should attend to team development during this stage, including individual development of strengths and interpersonal skill development.

A final stage, *adjourning*, was added by Tuckman to the original Team Development Model in the 1970s. Although this stage may not be applicable to ongoing teams, attendance to some leadership tasks during this stage is important for teams that are brought together for a specific mission. During the *adjourning* stage, the team has completed its work and the mission is completed. They have met their goals, and have evaluated not only the outcomes of their work together toward their goals, but have evaluated the team processes, and how they facilitated their work together.

EXEMPLAR FOR STAGES OF TEAM DEVELOPMENT

Consider the team we met earlier in this chapter, whose mission was to become "the provider of choice in our region because of the quality of care we provide supported by the implementation of a Professional Practice Model." The team was tasked with the development and implementation of a Professional Practice Model, and was made up of stakeholders from a variety of departments. As the team came together and began its work, consider how Tuckman's Stages of Team Development are evident in their work together:

> The Professional Practice Model team was appointed and the team leader was designated. The team leader brought the team together and guided them through the process of developing their team charter, their mission, vision, and ground rules for team operation (*Forming*). As the team began its work, conflict about how the work would be undertaken ensued. Because the team had not decided about how they would approach decisions, several opposing factions with differing ideas for how to approach the work began working independently of the team. One team member suggested that perhaps the team leader might not be the best equipped to lead the team in this effort. Team meetings were chaotic, and ground rules were inconsistently applied (*Storming*). Finally, the team leader called a meeting and brought the team together around its team vision, and the team re-affirmed its ground rules and decided that decisions would be made using a consensus process. Common ground among the opposing factions was found. The team became more settled, and began to trust one another. The team leader functioned as a facilitator for the team's work, and felt as if she didn't need to guide the team in one direction or another, that the team was functioning together and could guide itself reliably. The team made decisions easily, and consensus around a Professional Practice Model that would work for their organization was reached (*Norming*).

The team began to work toward a plan for implementation of the model in their organization, considering how the entire system would be impacted by the change. The larger environment was taken into consideration as they planned the implementation and evaluation of the Professional Practice Model (*Performing*). After about a year and a half of working together, the team was able to disband. The team members role-modeled support of the Professional Practice Model, having successfully implemented the model, and navigated the environment for a successful change in the organization (*Adjourning*).

SUMMARY AND NEXT STEPS

This chapter can help a team leader develop the ideal environment within which the team can function at a high level. The environment is critical to the success of the work of a team and team leaders can create the environment for success by purposefully thinking through the necessary balance of external supports and internal structures to facilitate a team's work. Teams and their leaders cannot underestimate the impact of professionalism, mutual understanding among team members, and relational coordination as external environmental factors impacting the work of a team. Likewise, through creating a few internal team structures, such as a team charter, mission and vision, goals, ground rules, methods to handle conflict, and transparency, the environment can be created to facilitate accomplishment of the team's goals. Finally, an understanding of the normal trajectory of team development cannot only assist a team in understanding the natural course of a team's growth, but can allow members to navigate the rocky times and celebrate their successes. In the next chapters, we will focus on the external environment that the team must work within for success, and will develop skill in developing perspectives about organizations that can influence how a team approaches its work.

QUESTIONS FOR THOUGHT

1. Apply the professionalism inventory to your team. In which areas are your strengths as a team? Which areas do you need to commit to work on for your team's professionalism to be improved?
2. Analyze your team for the presence of the concepts of relational coordination, including relationships and communication. How can your team improve?

3. Assess the utility of various technology applications for enhancing sharing of team information.
4. Develop a team charter for an existing or future team. How can a team charter facilitate your success as a team?
5. Develop a plan to enhance the transparency of your team's work within your organization. What avenues are present in your organization for sharing the work of the team?
6. Analyze where your team is developmentally based on Tuckman's stages of team development. Provide examples of how your team has behaved during a variety of stages of its development.

Nursing and Health Care Teams in Action

FIVE

Working as a Team Within the Nursing and Health Care Organization

The ratio of We's to I's is the best indicator of the development of a team.
—Lewis B. Ergen

LEARNING OBJECTIVES

1. Conduct an organizational analysis, including an assessment of organizational culture, structures and communication patterns, image, and politics.
2. Describe how organizational analysis can be used by teams to facilitate success.
3. Analyze the impact of organizational leadership on team success.
4. Identify mechanisms for communication both inside and outside of the organization that teams might use to facilitate success.

How many times have we stopped to really think about how our organizations work? One of the key factors in the success of a team is the team's ability to work within its organization to collaboratively accomplish a shared mission and purpose. To be successful, team leaders and members must get to know their organization in depth, cultivating an understanding of organizational culture and influences, insights into organizational leadership, and patterns of organizational behavior. The savvy and successful team will use these organizational perspectives to influence the organization and facilitate change.

STRATEGIC ORGANIZATIONAL ANALYSIS FOR TEAM SUCCESS

Key leadership competencies often cited in the health care, business, and other literature include self-knowledge, an awareness of how others behave in a variety of situations, an understanding of the dynamics of groups, and knowledge of how to facilitate change. None of these competencies can be practiced in isolation outside of an organizational system. Consequently, an analysis of organizational culture, structures and communication patterns, image, and politics can only enhance the team's strategic ability to lead change in its organization.

ORGANIZATIONAL CULTURE

Organizational culture is a "set of values that helps an organization's employees understand which actions are considered acceptable and which actions are considered unacceptable" (Griffin & Moorhead, 2011, p. 500). Values are sometimes less than obvious within an organization, so keen observers will analyze a variety of sources to gain insights into those values. In fact, organizational culture has been described as elements that operate on a less than conscious level. Schein (1990) defined culture in an organization as "as a pattern of basic assumptions, invented, discovered, or developed by a given group, as it learns to cope with its problems of external adaptation and internal integration, that has worked well enough to be considered valid and, therefore is to be taught to new members as the correct way to perceive, think, and feel in relation to those problems" (p. 111). So, culture includes deeply held assumptions and beliefs that form the basis of the organization's view of itself and the environment in which it exists. Organizational culture reflects long-held traditions, history, and philosophy, all of which help to influence current actions and responses. Organizational culture pervades all aspects of the work environment.

Organizational culture has been studied in a variety of industries. Some common observations of organizational culture include increased success in corporations with strong organizational cultures. Kotter and Heskett (2011) have reported that in strong corporate cultures, all managers share a set of similar values and methods for doing business. These values are adopted quickly by new employees. Organizations with strong cultures are usually seen by outsiders as having a certain way of doing things, or "style." These organizations with strong cultures make their values obvious in their mission, and most of the organization is "mission driven," encouraged to live those values. These cultures typically enjoy long-term success. Often cited as one of the strongest examples of corporate culture is Toyota; its culture is sometimes called "The Toyota Way." "The Toyota Way" embodies the culture of the Japanese automobile manufacturer and has five elements that have contributed to the company's success:

1. *Kaizen* is the Japanese process of continuous improvement. Toyota employees come to work every day with a philosophy that they will strive to be a little better at whatever it is they are doing than they were the previous day.

2. *Genchi genbutsu* is a Japanese phrase that means "go to the source." Employees must find the facts about issues because it is easier to build consensus around arguments that are well supported with facts rather than speculation. The culture also dictates that employees must go to the source of the problem for information. *Genchi genbutsu* emphasizes fully defining the problem before attempting to find solutions.

3. *Challenge* is a key element of Toyota's corporate structure. Toyota employees are encouraged to see problems as a way to help them to improve their performance, not as impeding their progress.

4. *Teamwork* is not only a key element of the Toyota corporate culture, but it also is an area in which Toyota invests deeply. Teamwork in this culture means putting the company's interests before those of the individual, and sharing knowledge with others in the team.

5. *Respect* for other people is the final key element in Toyota's culture. Respect is not just for others as people but for their skills and the knowledge and expertise they hold because of their position in the company. The Toyota culture values differences of opinion expressed respectfully and based on differing knowledge and expertise. Toyota believes that if two people always agree, one of them is superfluous ("Inculcating Culture," 2006).

Toyota demonstrates attributes of many strong successful organizational cultures. These strong cultures quite simply rely on integrating quality, support, and ownership of problems into their culture at every level.

Numerous studies over the past 20 years relate nursing care to organizational culture and quality. For instance, hospitals known to be "good places to work" have a lower mortality rate for older adults (Aiken, Smith, & Lake, 1994). A culture that is supportive of change has been found to be directly related to patient satisfaction (Caldwell et al., 2008). Organizational support for staff is known to affect job satisfaction and burnout, which impact quality of care (Aiken, Clarke, & Sloane, 2002; Aiken, Clarke, Sloane, Sochalski, & Silber, 2002). This has led to a call for a better understanding of organizational context and culture and its relationship to quality (Aiken, Sochalski, & Lake, 1997). Organizational culture has also been linked to safety, and the creation of a safety culture is a key part of improving patient and staff safety (Clark, 2002; Clarke, Sloane, & Aiken, 2002; Firth-Cozens, 2001; Gillies, Shortell, Casalino, Robinson, & Rundall, 2003; Mawji et al., 2002). Tzeng, Ketefian, and Redman (2002) investigated the relationship among staff nurses' assessment of organizational culture, job satisfaction, and inpatient satisfaction with nursing care. They found that strength of organizational culture predicted job satisfaction and job satisfaction predicted patient satisfaction.

How Do We Assess Organizational Culture?

Evidence of organizational culture can be explicit or implicit. Teams can use a variety of methods to uncover a clear picture of their organizational culture. Explicit evidence of organizational culture includes written organizational mission statements, vision statements, stated core values and purpose, policies, procedures, and the organizational chart. These items provide insight into the structure, accepted communication channels, and relationships among people and departments. Implicit evidence of culture often eludes verbal description, but is equally as important in strategic analysis of the organization. Implicit cultural cues are manifested informally in unwritten expectations and rules regarding patterns of communication, traditions, and measures of success.

Many frameworks for analyzing organizational culture have been developed since the early 1980s, when interest in the evaluation of organizational culture became popular among management experts. Characteristics of organizational culture have been identified and serve as a means for assessment of culture. For a team that is trying to assess its organizational culture to support planning for team success, a simple framework that analyzes image, deportment, status symbols and rewards, environment and ambience, communication, meetings, rites and rituals, and finally sacred cows could be effective. The following table of questions can serve as a tool for teams to use in their own organizational analysis (Table 5.1).

Another framework of characteristics of organizational culture expands upon the simpler framework noted above. The framework posited by Robbins and Judge (2012) includes the concepts of member

TABLE 5.1
Organizational Culture: Questions for Thought

CHARACTERISTIC OF ORGANIZATIONAL CULTURE	QUESTIONS FOR THOUGHT
Organizational image	How does the organization wish to be perceived? Are funds spent to create this image? How does the public get access to the organization? Is community involvement expected of employees? Is the organization seen as stable? Flexible? High performing?
Deportment	Is there an accepted way to present oneself in the organization? Does it matter who you associate with, or does it depend on your position? Do employees use first names with each other? Does it depend on job rank?
Status symbols and rewards	Are there any special symbols of status such as space, titles? Are there committees, projects, events only available to certain groups? How are people rewarded? What rewards are coveted?
Environment and ambience	Is there a company color scheme? Are there company symbols? Is there a company slogan, and where does it appear?
Communication	What is the norm for communication—verbal or written? Are written communications formal or informal? Are there company newsletters, bulletin boards, magazines? What is their purpose—recognition, information, both? How does important information flow in the organization? Top-down or bottom-up? Can the chain of command be circumvented? For what purpose? Where does important communication occur? In meetings, in the hallway, at social functions, away from the place of business?
Meetings	Do meetings have agendas? Who develops the agenda? Is it followed? Is discussion allowed at meetings? Are there unwritten rules about who speaks at meetings?
Rites and rituals	How does orientation to the organization occur? How does recognition occur in the organization? Are there established rituals that must be followed?
Sacred cows	Are there heroes (living or dead) in the organization who are honored and revered? Are there myths about the organization that are perpetuated? Are there any subjects or ideas that are taboo?

identity, group emphasis, people focus, unit integration, control, risk tolerance, reward criteria, conflict tolerance, means–end orientation, and open system focus. This framework can help develop insight for a team seeking greater depth of understanding of its organization's culture, and may also help them to plan for success. Again, the savvy team will use insights gained in studying the organization with this framework to guide planning, avoid potential organizational barriers, and secure support and resources needed for success. *Member identity* refers to how much individuals identify with the organization as a whole rather than their job, role, or profession. *Group emphasis* refers to the extent to which work in the organization is organized around groups or teams, rather than about individuals. *People focus* is the extent to which decision making in the organization takes into account the impact of the outcomes of those decisions on people in the organization. *Unit integration* is the extent to which departments, units, and teams are encouraged to coordinate and collaborate with each other. *Control* refers to the degree to which the organization uses policies, rules, and close supervision to manage the behavior and outputs of staff. *Risk tolerance* is the degree to which members of the organization are encouraged and supported in innovating and taking risks. *Reward criteria* is the degree to which rewards, including salary enhancement and promotions, are provided based on performance, rather than seniority, favoritism, nepotism, or other nonperformance-related factors. *Conflict tolerance* is the degree to which the organization encourages the open expression of concerns, conflicts, and criticism. *Means–End orientation* refers to the degree to which the organization's leadership focuses on outcomes rather than processes used to achieve outcomes. Finally, *Open systems focus* is the extent to which the organization is responsive to trends and events that occur externally to the organization. Table 5.2 poses key questions for thought for a team using this framework to gain insights into organizational culture.

Typologies or models of organizational culture have led to more formal, research-based assessment tools that can be used by a team to study its culture and identify methods for success. A common model and its associated measurement tools have been developed by Cameron and Quinn (2011). Cameron and Quinn have developed the Organizational Culture Assessment Instrument (OCAI) (see www.ocai-online.com for an online version of the instrument). Research with a variety of organizations led to the development of the Competing Values Framework (Quinn & Rohrbaugh, 1981). The OCAI consists of four competing values that correspond to four types of organizational

TABLE 5.2

Ten Characteristics of Organizational Culture: Questions for Thought

CHARACTERISTIC	QUESTIONS FOR THOUGHT
Member identity	Do employees identify with the whole organization? Do members of the organization compete with each other for recognition? Does the organization expend resources to influence organizational identity by its employees?
Group emphasis	Are work activities organized around groups? Individuals? Do rewards recognize individuals or groups?
People focus	Do management decisions consider the impact of those decisions on employees? Are unintended consequences of decisions studied?
Unit integration	Is work organized in a coordinated way? Are there ample opportunities for units to share their work? Collaborate? Does the organizational structure/reporting structure facilitate collaboration? Do communication systems exist to support collaboration?
Control	Are guidelines for professional behavior the norm? Are rules in place to control employee behavior? Is stringent adherence to rules the norm?
Risk tolerance	Are employees encouraged to be creative? Innovative? Initiate change? Are there examples of risk taking in the organization? Is risk taking rewarded? Are mistakes tolerated?
Reward criteria	Are rewards based upon performance? Is merit a basis for salary increase? Are rewards given to individuals or groups?
Conflict tolerance	Are conflicts of opinion and discussion of opposing views tolerated? Is constructive criticism encouraged? Are controversial issues discussed in an open format?
Means–end orientation	Is the outcome praised regardless of the process? Does the organization analyze processes for improvement? Are system issues attended to even if outcomes are positive?
Open system focus	How does the organization stay apprised of external trends? Is there evidence of responsiveness to external environments?

culture. Cameron and Quinn believe that all organizations have a mix of the four types of organizational culture, with most organizations having a dominant culture style. Although Cameron and Quinn believe that there are no "best" organizational cultures, a specific type of culture may be best in specific situations, and members of the organization can use the culture to their advantage in facilitating success. The four culture types identified by Cameron and Quinn and measured in the OCAI are:

1. *The Clan Culture:* In this culture, commitment is high. The culture feels like a family. People share information, and are involved in each other's lives. Organizational leaders are seen as mentors and sometimes as parent figures. Loyalty and tradition are high. The organization invests in cohesion, morale, and hence, its people. Empowerment of others is an essential value. Success is defined by how customer's concerns are met. The clan culture places a great deal of emphasis on teamwork, consensus, and collaboration to meet goals.
2. *The Adhocracy Culture:* In this culture, risk taking and creativity are valued. The culture is buzzing with creativity and an entrepreneurial spirit. Organizational leaders are risk takers, innovators, and sometimes mavericks. The highest value of the organization is innovation and creativity. The organization strives to lead and be at the cutting edge in its work. The organization is extremely agile and responds quickly to environmental trends.
3. *The Market Culture:* In this culture, the bottom line is outcomes and results. Measurable goals and outcomes drive actions. Employees are competitive and goal oriented. Leaders are producers and competitors. The emphasis is always placed on winning. High value is placed on the organization's reputation.
4. *The Hierarchy Culture:* In this culture, policies and procedures guide actions. Structure is high. Leaders are efficient and organized. The emphasis of the organization is on stability and smooth performance. The organization demands predictability.

Each of these cultures is measured along two dimensions in the OCAI, that of internal focus and integration versus external focus and differentiation, and flexibility and discretion versus stability and control. Results from the completion of this questionnaire provide a team with a look at the dominant culture, as well as organizational preferences and trends in the competing value dimensions (Figure 5.1).

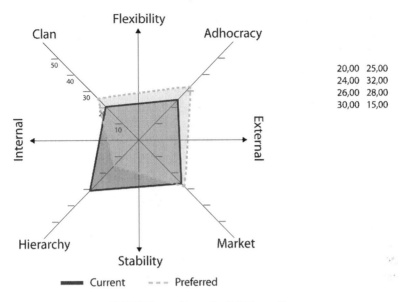

FIGURE 5.1 Sample OCAI profile.

Note: Numbers correspond to current and preferred culture grid coordinates beginning with clan culture and progressing in a clockwise fashion.

Source: Reprinted with permission from ocai-online.com.

O'Reilly, Chatman, and Caldwell (1991) have developed a model based on the belief that cultures can be distinguished by values that are reinforced within organizations. Their Organizational Profile Model (OCP) is a self-reporting tool that includes seven categories of organizational characteristics—Innovation, Stability, Respect for People, Outcome Orientation, Attention to Detail, Team Orientation, and Aggressiveness. This model was originally designed to assess person–organization fit, and has been used to measure the potential fit of applicants for a certain organization, but could also be used to guide the selection of team members who "fit" the organizational culture. O'Reilly and colleagues documented that person–organization fit predicts job satisfaction and organizational commitment a year after fit was measured and actual turnover after 2 years. This instrument was later revised by Cable and Judge (1997) for ease of use (see www.timothy-judge.com/OCP.htm for an online version of the revised instrument).

Although the two instruments referenced here are the most commonly cited organizational culture assessment inventories, Scott and colleagues (2003a, 2003b) published an excellent review of 13 organizational culture inventories (including the OCAI and OCP) that have the potential to be used in health care settings. In their review, they included an examination of the cultural dimensions addressed in each instrument, the number of items for each questionnaire, the measurement scale, examples of studies that used the tool, key properties of the instrument such as reliability and validity, and its strengths and limitations. Teams who need specific or more in-depth cultural assessment instruments may want to access these tools. Scott and colleagues' analysis can be found online at www.ncbi.nlm.nih.gov/pmc/articles/ PMC1360923/#b24. Reviews of reliability and validity may be especially helpful for teams using the instruments for a rigorous evaluation of culture and culture change in the organization. Scott and colleagues (2003a, 2003b) suggest that the choice of instruments be guided by how the team conceptualizes organizational culture, the purpose of the use of the instrument, the intended use of the results, and the availability of resources for purchase, administration, and evaluation of results.

Types of Cultures

Charles Handy, in his book *Gods of Management* (1995), describes four types of cultures, each with distinct characteristics. Many of these characteristics are played out in the models described earlier. Handy proposes that there are four types of cultures: *power, task, person,* and *role.*

1. *Power (or Club) Culture:* There are some organizations in which the power is centralized, and only those who hold power are authorized to make decisions. In this type of culture, the competencies of the leader are keys to organizational success as the leader remains the major decision maker.
2. *Task Culture:* Organizations in which teams are formed to achieve the organizational goals follow the task culture. Individuals with common interests and expertise form teams. Power and influence are based on expertise. In such a culture, every team member has to contribute equally and accomplish tasks using the collective expertise of the team. Control issues can be a detriment to the successful operation of the organization in this culture.
3. *Person (or Existential) Culture:* In a person culture, the emphasis is on individuals. Individual specialization and expertise are essential. Structures are developed to support the specialist. A problem with this type of culture is a lack of loyalty to the organization, with attrition high in times of organizational flux or challenge.
4. *Role Culture:* Role culture is a culture in which the emphasis is on roles rather than individuals. This culture is fairly typical of large

bureaucracies. In a role culture, employees are selected based on their experience, education, and specialization. Every individual is accountable for his or her role, and takes ownership of the work assigned. Power comes with responsibility and outcomes.

ORGANIZATIONAL STRUCTURE

Closely aligned with organizational culture, organizational structure is the framework within which an organization arranges its lines of authority and communication, and delineates duties and obligations (Marion, 2001). Organizational structure determines the manner in which information flows among levels of the organization. Organizational structure also delineates how roles, power, and responsibilities are delegated, controlled, and coordinated. The most obvious demonstration of organizational structure is the organizational chart. A savvy team will understand how organizational structure can impact their success.

There are a number of organizational structures that have been adopted in health care organizations. Traditional organizational structures focus on the functions, or departments, within an organization. These structures have clearly defined lines of authority for all levels of management. These structures are sometimes called *hierarchical* structures, but frequently are called *line* and *line-and-staff* structures. The *line* structure is fairly flat with few departments, and is defined by a clear chain of command with final approval on decisions affecting the organization coming from the top down. The line structure is most often effective in small organizations, and in health care might be used in small primary care centers, long-term care settings, or sometimes in small single-specialty hospitals or clinics, like surgical centers. The president or chief executive officer (CEO) is close to the workers, and therefore can provide information and direction quickly, facilitating rapid decision making. *Line and staff* structures combine the flow of information from the line structure with staff departments that support the goals of the organization. In health care, this type of organization is commonly used in small hospitals, larger primary care settings, and sometimes in small public health departments. In this structure, line managers are responsible for the flow of information to their subordinates, and are accountable for the work of their subordinates in meeting the goals of the organization. Staff managers are responsible for activities that support the work of the organization. Activities such as purchasing, accounting, public relations and marketing, and education may be designated at the staff level. Line-and-staff managers have direct authority over their subordinates, but staff managers have no authority over line managers and their subordinates. Because of the layers inherent in a line and staff structure, decision making can be slow and will require the team to communicate and collaborate with multiple departments to initiate change. A less traditional organizational structure is known as the *matrix* structure. Organizations arranged according to projects are referred to as *matrix organizations*. In a matrix structure, employees are hired into a functional department but may work on projects managed by members of another department. Matrix organizations combine both vertical authority relationships (where employees report to their functional manager) and horizontal, or diagonal, work relationships (where employees report to their project supervisor for the length of the project). This type of structure is more complex; however, it is functional in achieving organizational goals. Although not explicitly cited as such, many health care organizations today function in a matrix structure out of necessity to achieve patient care and organizational goals. Interprofessional teams are a perfect example of the matrix model in action. Typically, team members are hired into a department (nursing, social work, pharmacy, etc.) and report to a manager or director in that department. However, the interprofessional team comes together around particular goals (typically patient or population driven) and works together to meet those goals. The interprofessional team members are accountable to the team leader, while also being held accountable for their performance by their departmental manager or director.

Any of these structures can also be characterized by the level of centralization of power within the structure. In a highly *centralized* structure, several layers of management maintain a high level of authority, typically the power to make decisions concerning activities and priorities of the organization. With a centralized structure, line-and-staff employees have limited authority to act without prior approval. This organizational structure tends to be described as "top-down" in which executives at the top communicate with middle managers, who then communicate with lower frontline managers, who then communicate with the staff. In a more *decentralized* structure, authority is placed at the level of frontline managers, eliminating multiple layers of bureaucracy, allowing more efficient flow of information, facilitating "bottom-up" communication, and supporting more rapid decision making. Authority for problem recognition and development of solutions is delegated to staff who have a greater span of control.

ORGANIZATIONAL IMAGE

Organizational image is a "holistic and vivid impression held by an individual or a particular group towards an organization and is a result of sense-making by the group *and* communication by the organization of a fabricated and projected picture of itself. Such communication by the organization occurs as top managers and corporate spokespersons orchestrate deliberate attempts to influence public impression" (Hatch & Schultz, 1997, p. 356). In his classic text, Gareth Morgan (2006) uses several metaphors to describe organizational image. Morgan uses the metaphors of *machine, organism, brain, social structure, political system, psychic prison, flux and transformation,* and *systems of domination* to describe organizational images. The *machine* image is one of an organization that strives to be sure that everyone in the organization has a job, and everyone performs that job, similar to a machine. Everyone in the organization is a "cog in the wheel." This is an image supported by classical management theory—each person in the organization can be managed in his or her "job." The *organism* image is one in which organizations put forth an image of adaptation to the environment. An organizational image similar to a *brain* is one in which the organization is seen as constantly processing information and learning. A *social* metaphor describes the organization as a social system with a distinct culture. The *political system* metaphor describes an organization in which interests and rights, power, authority, and alliances are the hallmarks of behavior. A negative metaphor of the organization as a *psychic prison* is used to describe an organization in which repression, denial, and other coping mechanisms are dominant. Finally, in *systems of domination*, force, exploitation, wielding of power, compliance, and alienation are common.

ORGANIZATIONAL POLITICS

When you hear the words "organizational politics," what comes to mind? Organizational politics, although usually carrying a negative connotation, is really just about the use of power and influence to meet goals. Who has power and influence, who gets power and influence, and how can we use power and influence to the advantage of our goals are the key questions for a team to ask. Interestingly, every member of an organization holds power and influence and makes decisions about how to wield that power and influence in order to either benefit himself or herself or the organization. Power and influence are not just centered at the top levels of an organization, regardless of organizational structure. Think about the staff nurse who purposefully develops a "work around" rather than working through the system to change a faulty process. That nurse has wielded power to influence the work of providing care to the patient. Whether positive or negative, the nurse has demonstrated power. A successful team will understand how power and influence, and hence politics, play out at every level of its organization, and will then negotiate within that structure of power and influence to navigate the organization.

USE OF STRATEGIC ORGANIZATIONAL ANALYSIS BY TEAMS

Every organizational culture works on different assumptions about behavior, power, and influence, how people communicate, learn, and are motivated. In every culture, change is initiated, accepted, and integrated in different ways. Team success is dependent upon a clear understanding of these factors in the organization, and then putting that knowledge to use in planning, implementing, and subsequently evaluating change. The following case example demonstrates how an understanding of organizational culture, structure, image, and politics worked to the advantage of one team.

> In a small critical access hospital in a rural area, leadership has noted an increase in the use of overtime on the nursing units. This increase has driven costs up, and has caused discontent among staff as they are increasingly being called upon to work longer hours. The CEO, who reports to the board of trustees, approaches the chief nursing officer (CNO) and tasks her to "solve the problem." The CNO puts together a team made up of the nurse managers from the three nursing units in this small hospital to investigate the cause of the overtime problem, and to implement a solution.
>
> The team begins by examining all overtime over the last 6 months. They confirm that overtime costs have increased across the organization over the last 3 months. They note that beginning 3 months ago, there was an increase in staff across the hospital calling in sick for more than 1 day at a time, and that the average amount of time missed by staff during this period of time was 3 days. The nurse managers

realized that 4 months ago, a new Human Resources (HR) policy was put into place that allows staff to only have two "call ins" per year, and once they reach three "call ins," they are entered into the disciplinary process, with first a verbal, then written warning, and finally ending in termination. A "call in" is defined as any occurrence in which a staff member is absent from work. A single "call in" can occur for up to 3 days without being counted as an additional "call in." Staff had quickly identified that if they were "going to call in 1 day, they might as well call in for 3."

The team began to deliberate about how to solve this problem. Here is what they knew about their culture once they completed an organizational analysis.

1. Conflict is not tolerated. The image portrayed of the organization is one of a tight-knit family.
2. Rewards are public, but typically are "pats on the back" as opposed to tangible acknowledgments.
3. The organizational structure follows a line and staff model. Decisions are made based upon data. Decisions are made at the CEO and Board level, and impact and unintended consequences are rarely taken into account.
4. The HR director is a "sacred cow," having come up through the ranks of the organization, and is lauded as a "hometown hero." The CEO has an excellent working relationship with the HR director, but others in the organization do not.
5. The organization strives to be "the best place to work" for its small rural community.

How did the team use this information about their culture to influence a change in policy?

The team first recognized that criticism of the policy would not be tolerated, as it may also be seen as criticism of the HR director, and would likely lead to conflict. The team decided to use its understanding of the image of a tight-knit family, the reward system used in the organization, the vision of becoming the "best place to work," and knowledge that data drives decisions to plan their solution. The team undertook an employee satisfaction survey to find out what organizational components led to satisfaction and dissatisfaction. In addition, they began exit interviews with all staff leaving the organization to see whether organizational policy had an impact on their decisions. Armed with data that the "call in" policy was a major dissatisfier in their "family," and was causing the community to not want to work in this organization, the team went back to the CEO, provided these data, and proposed an alternate policy that worked on a reward rather than punishment system that could be piloted in the organization. They asked the CEO to support this policy with the HR director, using their understanding of not only the CEO's power but also the CEO's influence with the HR director, which could propel their ideas forward.

Although this assessment of organizational culture, structure, image, and politics may have taken a bit longer to accomplish than simply coming together as a team and deciding on a solution to a fairly simple problem, this team's success was based on careful planning using knowledge and respect of the organizational norms. The team strategically considered how to best lead change in the organization.

IMPACT OF ORGANIZATIONAL LEADERSHIP ON TEAMWORK

Leadership has a significant impact on all aspects of the organization. Culture, function, and structure are directly linked to organizational leadership through implicit support and explicit actions. Organizational leadership can facilitate or impede the work of a team. A careful analysis of leadership within any organization, as well as a plan for how to best work together with leadership, will serve any team well in reaching its ultimate goals. Montes, Moreno, and Morales (2005) found that supportive leadership encourages teamwork cohesion, learning, and innovation within an organization, in their study of over 200 businesses in Spain. Yun, Cox, Sims, and Salam (2007) studied leadership and its impact on team citizenship behavior, and found that there was a direct relationship between empowering and transformational leadership styles in an organization and the actions of teams. Given the strong documented impact of leadership in an organization on teams and their success, team leaders and members will want to analyze leadership styles in the organization and plan for how to best work with the leadership.

LEADERSHIP STYLES

On the basis of earlier work by other researchers, Yun and colleagues (2007) describe five leadership archetypes found in organizations. These include aversive, directive, transactional, transformational, and empowering leadership archetypes.

Aversive Leadership

Aversive leadership methods focus on punishment and reprimand. Leaders using aversive techniques will typically focus on weaknesses in their followers, poor outcomes of their work, or unacceptable actions. Intimidation techniques are commonly used by aversive leaders.

Directive Leadership

Directive leadership methods focus on issuing commands and instructions, and expecting follow through by followers. Directive leaders gain their authority from their position in the organization. They are highly decisive and commanding.

Transactional Leadership

Transactional leaders focus on relationships negotiated between themselves and their followers. Transactional leaders provide information about what is expected, and feedback about performance. They strategically provide rewards for positive outcomes.

Transformational Leadership

Transformational leaders have a vision that is clearly articulated, and they inspire others to perform to meet or exceed that vision. Charismatic influence motivates followers to go beyond their normal performance levels, to innovate, and to change the status quo.

Empowering Leadership

Empowering leaders focus on empowering others to "self-lead." Empowering leaders believe that every member of an organization has something to offer, and the role of the leader is to set up situations in which members can self-lead—using their talents to change the organization.

Consider these four leadership archetypes and their potential impact on a team. When teams recognize the leadership styles of those in their organization who have power or influence over their work, they can begin to plan how to work with those leaders to ensure success. For example, suppose a team is faced with a directive leader. The team will want to focus on seeking opportunities to hear the leader's instructions for action within the team. Because this type of leader expects followers to carry through on his or her directives, the team will be well served in seeking input and direction from this leader. Similarly, with a transactional leader, the team will want to have a rational exchange with the leader while negotiating expectations for performance, and allowing plenty of opportunities for the leader to provide the team feedback on its performance. On the other hand, with a transformational leader, the team will want to have adequate time to listen to the vision of the leader, to seek out encouragement from this leader for examining and changing the status quo. Cultivating an understanding of the leadership styles of organizational leaders will only enhance the team's planning for success within the organization. Taking the time to match team strategies to leadership styles within the organization will serve the team well in their work.

COMMUNICATION OF INFORMATION WITHIN AND OUTSIDE OF THE ORGANIZATION

Much of the work done by teams depends on clear and frequent communication. How information is communicated outside of the team both within and outside of the organization is closely related to the organizational culture, structure, and leadership styles within the organization. Using knowledge of the organization in planning communication strategies will set up the team for success.

Communication Within the Organization

There will be many opportunities for teams to communicate about their work within an organization. Strategically planning how that communication occurs should be a team priority. Taking time at each team meeting to discuss communication strategies will allow the team to be purposeful in its communication, communicating the right information, in the right format, at the right time, and to the right groups or individuals. Strategic communication can occur at all times during a team's work together. Particular opportunities for communication are suggested in the text that follows.

Communication of team formation: Consider how as a team you might communicate the formation of your team, your mission, and even your charter to others within the organization. Communication at the outset of your work with those inside the organization who might have an interest in your work can help to garner additional support for your team, and can increase transparency and trust within the organization. Who communicates the team's formation is a question of organizational culture and norms, and teams should consider the appropriate person to announce the team's formation prior to doing so themselves. Discussions with leaders, sponsors, and mentors will allow the team to come up with an appropriate communication plan at this time.

Communication of team strategies and barriers: Selective release of strategies being used in the work of the team may also garner support and/or resources for the team. As others within the organization become excited about the potential of the team's work, resources may be offered that were previously unrecognized. In addition, communication during the work of the team may allow linkages to be made with the work of other individuals and teams within the organization. Similarly, communication of barriers being experienced by teams may bring attention to organizational structures or functions that are barriers to other progress as well. Creative solutions to similar barriers experienced by others in the organization may also be offered. Again, teams will want to carefully consider organizational culture, norms, and structure as well as leadership styles when strategizing about how to release information at this time. Certainly, the wise team will be especially contemplative when considering how and with whom to communicate about organizational barriers to their success. No team wants to be caught in the political crossfire by communicating at the wrong level of the organization about organizational pitfalls!

Communication of team products: Probably the most crucial time for communication is at the point of roll out of the results of the team's work and its products. Especially if the team's work is high stakes, the plan for communication of the product will need to be especially well thought out. Using knowledge of change, of communication strategies with small and large groups, and rolling out large-scale initiatives will be helpful to a team planning to communicate its products. Consultation with crucial stakeholders in the process will be a necessity. Working with leadership, team sponsors, and mentors will continue to be essential in developing a communication plan. Again, considering organizational culture, structure, climate, and politics will be helpful in making decisions about timing of communication, formats, forums, and spokespersons for communication.

Communication within organizations can also take advantage of multiple formats. Websites, e-newsletters, e-mails, e-mail blasts, and printed newsletters may be a few of the written methods of communication available within the organization. In addition, in-person communication at in-house forums, committee meetings, town hall meetings, or staff meetings may be appropriate. The most important consideration for the team in selecting a method of communication is the appropriateness of the method to the message of the product and to organizational culture, norms, and politics.

Communication Outside of the Organization

Some teams may find themselves needing to communicate their work outside of the organization. Communication outside of the organization is indicated when the results of the team's work will have an impact on those outside of the organization, when the work has the potential for transforming the way care is provided or business is carried out, or when the need for additional resources is recognized as being sought outside of the organization.

Communicating work outside of the organization is typically more complicated than communicating inside of the organization. Because those outside of the organization, including customers, patients, families, donors, funders, and the press, may know little about what has led to the work of the team, clarity of background and purpose of the team's work are essential. Teams may use their skill in storytelling to make an impact on those outside of the organization with whom they are communicating. Messaging about changes to the way care is being provided and/or business is being conducted must also be extremely clear. If communicating with potential funders, teams will want to include how their work matches to the mission of the funding agency, in addition to how it fits into the bigger picture of the organization. Teams may want to call on experts within the organization to help them craft their messages for communication outside of the organization, including marketing experts, grant writers, or public relations staff. Regardless of how the messages to be communicated outside of the organization are crafted by the team, the team will need to continually assess how those messages match with the organization's culture and external image.

SUMMARY AND NEXT STEPS

A team's ability to work within the organization to collaboratively accomplish a shared mission and purpose is essential to success. By understanding its organization in depth, cultivating an understanding of organizational culture and influences, developing insights into organizational leadership and patterns of organizational behavior, the team can develop strategies that are consistent with organizational norms. The team will use these organizational insights to influence the organization and facilitate change through its work. In the next chapters, we will analyze how a team can successfully work together to share information, plan its work, and manage change in the organization.

QUESTIONS FOR THOUGHT

1. Describe the culture of the organization in which your team functions. How have implicit or explicit elements of the organizational culture informed the work of your team? How have they hindered the work of your team? How can leaders use knowledge of the organizational culture to facilitate team success?
2. Analyze the primary leadership styles evident in the leadership in your organization. How have these leadership styles impacted the work of your team? How can you use your understanding of leadership styles to enhance the work of the team?
3. Develop a communication plan for the work of a team in your organization. What avenues exist for communication of the process of your work? What avenues exist for communication of the products of your work?
4. Consider how you might communicate the work of your team to a potential funder of your work. How can you craft your communication so as to be consistent with your organization's mission and vision for the future?

SIX

Planning for Nursing and Health Care Team and Partnership Success

Big thinking precedes great achievement.
    —*Wilford Peterson*

LEARNING OBJECTIVES

1. Define the elements of a successful team meeting.
2. Identify methods for facilitating full team participation in team meetings.
3. Describe methods for communication of team meeting results.
4. Develop a structure for team project planning.
5. Understand the key elements of project evaluation.
6. Apply change theory to the work of teams.

Success does not just happen. It takes careful planning. To ensure success, any team or partnership will spend most of its time carefully planning approaches to problems, issues, or challenges. Careful planning will allow all team members and partners to have input into the team's strategies, and will pay off in the long term by decreasing implementation problems. This chapter addresses how a successful team structures team meetings, plans approaches to team challenges, uses existing tools for project or program planning, and manages change.

TEAM MEETINGS

Few of us would say that we enjoy meetings, whether as leaders or participants. Too often, meetings seem to have little focus and even less purpose. But, if you have ever been a part of a "great meeting," you recognize the difference. Planning and design are what lead to a great meeting. Knowledge of your team and partners, their personalities, the organizational culture, communication patterns, and a blueprint for your meeting will serve you well in moving toward productive team meetings.

In their primer *Anatomy of Great Meetings*, the 3M Company (1998) suggests that people meet for a variety of reasons, including presentation of information, collaboration, review, evaluation, discussion, problem solving, and decision making. But 3M also points out that people also meet for social reasons, such as the need to belong, achieve, and make an impact, and to build a common reality. Further, in order for tasks to be accomplished in meetings, social needs must also be met and vice versa. So, just what makes a successful team or partnership meeting?

In planning a successful meeting, leaders will plan both process and content. Meeting content will address the tasks that the team would like to accomplish, but meeting process will address the social needs of the team. Savvy team leaders will begin meetings by addressing social needs. With new teams, activities to meet social needs might include having each member talk briefly about who he or she is, what he or she does, and why he or she is attending the meeting. Meeting "icebreakers" are common ways to meet social needs while allowing team members to learn more about each other in the process. Hundreds of "ice breakers" are available in the literature and found on the web. For some great free ideas, you might visit the website of Team Building USA, at www.teambuildingusa.com/business-meeting-icebreakers.

Icebreakers should always have a purpose. Team leaders using icebreakers should be sure to match the icebreaker to the desired outcome of the exercise. For instance, in early team meetings, icebreakers that revolve around getting to know each other better, or establishing group norms would be most appropriate. A popular icebreaker to get to know each other is to interview a partner and then have the partner introduce the person he or she interviewed to the group. Suggested questions might be "tell me something no one knows about you," or "what is your favorite thing to do in your free time?" Connections among team members can be revealed by the answers to these questions in ways that would never be found with more traditional introduction methods. In a recent nursing leadership meeting, during an icebreaker two nurse leaders found that they had both served as mission nurses in the same town in South

America. Instant and lasting connections were made between these two nurses. Imagine what similar experiences can do for your team.

More established teams use icebreakers or games to knock down barriers within teams, to deal with issues around team participation, or to address resistance to change. A popular icebreaker in one team leadership program is the "build a vehicle exercise" in which teams are given a variety of items found in a local home improvement store, for instance, a 24 in. × 24 in. piece of plywood, clothesline, duct tape, plastic painting tarps, tubing, and so on, and are challenged to build a vehicle that will carry a team member across the room in a race against other teams. Secretly, the facilitator gives some team members roles to fulfill. One member is told to disengage completely, and under no circumstances to talk to the other team members. Another member is told to argue about every idea that is presented. Still another team member is told to agree with everything and to just want to get the project finished. In some teams, one member is told to take over from the team leader at every opportunity. The facilitator makes rounds during the exercise, encouraging the teams to explain what they are observing among their team members. After a race occurs and a winner is "crowned," the facilitator debriefs the teams with questions such as "What did you do about the team member who disengaged?" and "Did you feel that you wasted valuable time trying to engage them?" and to the leader, "How did you respond to the team member who wanted to be the leader?" Table 6.1 contains some additional potential debriefing questions, concepts to remember, and team strategies for success for this exercise.

During debriefing, teams share their strategies for overcoming team issues with each other, and discuss the value and danger of specific strategies. Team members are encouraged to use their team norms or ground rules to develop strategies for how to deal with these types of issues in actual team situations. This icebreaker obviously takes a significant amount of time; be sure that any icebreaker chosen to meet social needs during a meeting is the right length as compared to the time allotted for the meeting. In addition, be sure that as a team leader you are prepared not only to facilitate the icebreaker but to debrief it as well.

Team leaders may also strive to make connections among team members by telling stories about why the team exists. Storytelling is a powerful way to draw team members in and to make the mission of the team personal and meaningful. People are wired to respond to stories. From early childhood, we all identify with storytelling as a way to make connections. Individual stories are much more significant in

TABLE 6.1
Build-a-Vehicle Debriefing Questions

DEBRIEFING QUESTIONS	CONCEPTS TO STRESS	TEAM STRATEGIES FOR SUCCESS
How did your team come together around your mission?	Shared mission is essential to team success.	Take time at the beginning of the team's work together and periodically thereafter to be sure everyone understands and agrees to the mission of the team.
How did you use the skills of all team members to your team's advantage?	Diversity of team members adds strength to any team. Working from strengths will enhance the team's performance.	Allow team members to describe their strengths, or use a systematic assessment of strengths and share with the team. Purposefully plan to use those strengths in the work of the team.
Were all team members engaged? If not, how did the team respond to the disengaged member?	Team members' levels of engagement will differ during the life of a team. How team members react to differing levels of engagement may impact team accomplishments.	Plan for differing levels of engagement by discussing limits on time or output with all team members from the outset of the team's work together, and integrat those limitations into the plan for the team's work. Avoid focusing on team members who are less productive at certain times in the life cycle of the team, as this will take time and energy away from the team's goals.
Were there power struggles within the team? If so, how were they handled?	Power struggles are inevitable in teams, especially in their early stages of development. The leader's response to these struggles will impact future team success.	Take time to delineate roles and responsibilities of team members. As the team grows and matures, revisit roles and responsibilities as needed. Understand that as a team develops, team members become more autonomous. Leaders move from directors of activities, to facilitators of team success.
How did the team deal with conflict?	Conflict is inevitable in any relationship. Having a plan to deal with conflict within the team increases the productivity of the team.	When setting team ground rules, discuss how the team prefers to deal with conflict. Honor the commitment to the ground rules by dealing with conflict promptly and appropriately.

meeting social connection needs than data, so team leaders can use stories to help to transition from meeting social needs to moving to content or tasks of the meeting. Good storytellers will personalize their stories and ground them in the work of the team. A team working on patient handoffs might be tempted to move directly into data about the errors that occur during handoffs. This approach depersonalizes the issue that the team is working on, and can serve to distance the team from the importance of the problem. However, a team leader who begins a meeting telling a significant story of a handoff success or failure can help to ground the team, remind members of the reason they exist, and connect to the problem in a different way.

Once social process needs have been met, the team must move into the structure and content of the meeting. There are many different types of meetings, and the structure of the meeting should match the purpose. Typical meeting types are:

- Problem solving
- Decision making
- Strategic
- Planning
- Informational
- Feedback and evaluation
- Combination

Team meetings should be focused, transparent, and efficient, regardless of type. Team leaders should consider the culture of the organization regarding the formality of the meeting content. However, an agenda is always appropriate, regardless of culture. Typical meeting agendas begin with a recap of past meetings, typically in the form of a review and acceptance of the minutes. Many teams find that rather than beginning with a minutes review, they begin by revisiting their accepted team mission, vision, and purpose. Some teams revisit their ground rules at each meeting. Reviewing these agreed-upon items at the beginning of each meeting sets the stage for all subsequent discussions during the meeting, which can then be related back to the mission and purpose of the team. A public health interagency team charged with developing a statewide plan for immunization for an emerging infectious disease found this strategy especially successful as each team member came from a different organizational culture and was working on multiple teams and projects within their own agencies. This partnership's success in accomplishing his or her goals in a timely manner was attributed to their practice of reaffirming their mission and purpose at the beginning of every meeting, grounding everyone in the work to be done on the issue during that session and beyond. As one team member remarked, "Starting our meetings with our mission helped us to put aside our other hats and focus on the issue at hand."

Teams may also take an opportunity at the beginning of each meeting to reaffirm their team norms and ground rules. A team of nurse educators working on a new graduate curriculum reaffirmed their ground rules at each monthly curricular retreat. Ground rules and norms adopted by this group included listening with respect, speaking from the heart, and remembering what they never wanted to lose from the curriculum—quality, a focus on nursing perspectives, and an emphasis on evidence in practice. Finally, team members agreed that "once we come to agreement, while I may not completely agree with the result, I will not speak badly of our decisions when we leave the room." Team members appreciated the revisiting of the norms at the outset of each meeting, as these norms set the stage for the expected behaviors of the group at each meeting and beyond.

Once teams have revisited their mission and ground rules, the meeting structure becomes important. What meeting structures prove to be most effective for teams? In Chapter 1, we talked about Takeuchi and Nonaka (1986), who described the best teams they had seen around the world as self-organizing teams characterized by autonomy, transcendence, and cross-fertilization. These transformative teams became catalysts for innovation and organizational change. After reading Takeuchi and Nonaka's work, Shwaber and Sutherland (2011) developed a team process known as "scrum." Scrum is a rugby term that commonly denotes a group of players who congregate closely around the ball in order to move it forward toward the goal. What does rugby have to do with team processes in health care and other industries? The analogy is a strong one—teams in any situation must work together to meet goals. Although an entire process known as a "scrum" for product development has been developed (see www.scrum.org for more information), most pertinent to team meetings is what Shwaber and Sutherland (2011) call a "Daily Scrum." The Daily Scrum is a 15-minute time-limited meeting used for the team to synchronize activities and create a plan for its work for the next 24 hours. The team inspects the work since the last Daily Scrum and forecasts the work that could be done before the next one. The Daily Scrum is held at the same time and location each day to reduce complexity. Many teams chose to have their Daily Scrum first thing in the morning, prior to any interruptions. Others chose to do this as the last event of their day, to energize for the next day's work. Regardless of timing, during the meeting, each team member discusses the following three questions:

- What has been accomplished since the last meeting?
- What will be done before the next meeting?
- What obstacles are in the way?

The team uses the Daily Scrum to assess progress toward its goal. Shwaber and Sutherland (2011) believe that the Daily Scrum optimizes the probability that a team will meet its goals. At the end of the Daily Scrum, each team member should be able to explain how he or she intends to work together as a team to accomplish the agreed-upon goal. Shwaber and Sutherland (2011) hold that Daily Scrums "improve communications, eliminate other meetings, identify and remove impediments to development, highlight and promote quick decision-making, and improve the team's level of knowledge" (p. 11). Some scrum guidelines are found in Table 6.2.

Imagine implementing this 15-minute strategy each day or even every other day or once a week with your team. Even if you choose not to follow all of the Daily Scrum guidelines, the introduction of the three simple questions into every team meeting could be the solution to project backlogs, competing priorities, and loss of focus on the goal that your team needs.

Other effective team meeting structures are also available. White (1987) in his article about managing innovation adapted the Coverdale Organization's Systematic Approach (see www.coverdale.co.uk) to suggest a team structure that can be used for effective meetings. The steps in this process are as follows:

1. Define aims
2. Define end results
3. Gather information
4. Define what must be done
5. Take action
6. Review and evaluate

Depending upon progress toward the goal, meetings could be structured around all or a few of these steps. It is likely that early in your team's work, defining aims and end results or goals will take up a bulk of your time. Gathering information will include why current practices are in place, the important stakeholders in the process, and best practices from the literature and other organizations. Defining what must be done and how to accomplish the selected actions will

TABLE 6.2
Daily Scrum Guidelines

DAILY SCRUM GUIDELINE	PURPOSE
Choose a scrum leader	Maintain focus, enforce rules
Meeting should last no more than 15 to 30 minutes	Focus increased during short meetings
Hold meeting at the same time and place each day	Scrum becomes a routine part of daily work
Address the same three questions at each meeting: What has been accomplished since the last meeting? What will be done before the next meeting? What obstacles are in the way?	Assess progress and plan for next steps while recognizing and removing obstacles
Address any other issues that do not involve the three questions outside of the Daily Scrum	Keeps team focused on goal
Managers or any nonteam member may attend and observe the scrum, but cannot speak	Maintain purpose and focus among team members
If a manager or any other person assigns work to a team member that will throw the team's work off track, the scrum leader will excuse the team member from the work and negotiate reassignment of that work to a nonteam member	Allows individual team members to avoid conflicting priorities

Source: Adapted from: N.A. *Stay on track with scrum meetings*. (2004). Retrieved from www.effectivemeetings.com/teams/teamwork/scrum.asp

likely require brainstorming, followed by structured discussion and development of a plan of action. Once action is taken, team meetings should surround the process of implementation, a review of progress, and evaluation of results. Team leaders can use these elements to structure an effective team meeting agenda.

Software is also available to help with the effectiveness of team meetings. Most software for team meetings helps with brainstorming, prioritizing, surveying, voting, action planning, and documentation of results. There are many software programs available to serve these functions. A few are reviewed here, but a quick search of the web will reveal hundreds with different features to meet your needs. Some are free for download, others may appear as parts of other software packages already available in your institution. Some are proprietary and there is a license fee associated. Many have free demonstrations available. The team leader should evaluate the team's needs that can be met by software and then evaluate the products that meet those needs.

One software program that integrates all meeting functions is Facilitate Pro™ (www.facilitate.com). This program contains all of the features mentioned above, including survey functions, brainstorming via an online flip chart, all in a web-based platform. The program can be used synchronously in a meeting room, or can be used asynchronously as teams work together. A schematic of the capabilities of Facilitate Pro™ is found in Figure 6.1.

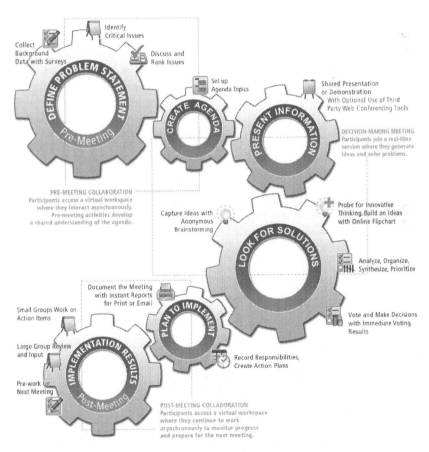

FIGURE 6.1 FacilitatePro™ capabilities.

Source: Reprinted from www.Facilitatepro.com. Copyright 2008. FacilitatePro.

MeetingSense® is another popular meeting management software program. A hosted software program (meaning data are saved on the MeetingSense server), MeetingSense® is capable of helping teams schedule meetings, capture information during meetings, assign action items, follow up with team members with meeting summaries and action item review, and track, collaborate, and manage team meeting information, action items, and files online in real time (www.meetingsense.com). A sample output from this software program is found in Figure 6.2.

Finally, regardless of the structure you choose, great team meetings start with a shared vision, shared values, engaged team members who respect and value each other's talents and skills, clear objectives, a clear understanding of obstacles to your success, and a clear system for follow up. If you have taken a lot of care in setting up the "right" team in the first place, the only challenge becomes making sure that the team understands the problems to be solved and has the information available to select and implement the best solutions. They

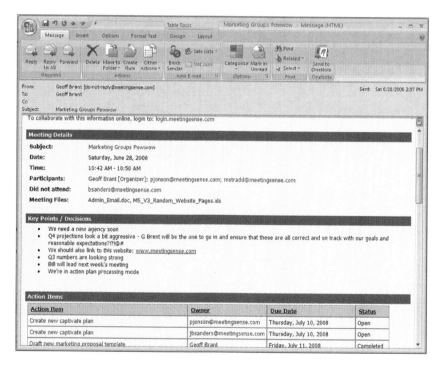

FIGURE 6.2 Meeting sense output sample.

Source: Reprinted with permission from www.meetingsense.com

will naturally create their own meetings and you as team leader will merely serve as a facilitator to the team's success!

ELEMENTS OF PROJECT PLANNING

Although meetings are where a team does its work, the structure of that work is typically around planning. The team can use project planning strategies to develop solutions for problems that range from simple to complex. Essentially, all project planning strategies contain some key elements that teams will want to take into account in their work. These include:

1. Problem identification
2. Hypothesis regarding causation
3. Intended outcomes
4. Objectives
5. Strategies
6. Resources required
7. Action steps
8. Evaluation

Problem Identification

During this phase of planning, the team will want to identify exactly what the problem is that the team is trying to address, or the need that they are trying to meet. Developing strategies to solve the right problem is a key to the teams', and eventually the organizations', success. Getting assumptions about problems out on the table will help to delineate the problem. Consider the following problem discussion by a recent doctor of nursing practice (DNP) graduate who is serving as the director of clinical practice in a professional organization representing home care agencies and her team. What problem is the DNP trying to influence her team to solve?

> We need to be thinking about how we can influence registered nurses in our home care agencies to use evidence upon which to base their practice. They need to understand the importance of using evidence to improve the outcomes for the vulnerable people they care for in their homes. But none of them want to even learn about evidence-based practice (EBP) by coming in for a day to learn about a model to use

evidence. If I could get them all to come into our building for even 6 hours, I could get them excited about EBP, and they will talk to and get to know each other and maybe we can cut down on the animosity among different agencies that is really affecting patient care.

Perhaps in this case, the real problem is animosity among different agencies and its impact on patient care, and not the need for education around EBP. Would the goals and strategies and potential outcomes look very different depending on which of these two problems the team is trying to solve? Of course they would. How can a team get to the real problem in its planning process? First, in-depth discussions about the problem will help. Getting a variety of perspectives about the problem will also assist the team. A more formal and fun way to try to identify what the problem is that the team needs to address is called the *Ladder of Inference.* The Ladder of Inference (sometimes called the *Process of Abstraction*) is a technique that was first put forward by organizational psychologist Chris Argyris and used by Peter Senge in *The Fifth Discipline: The Art and Practice of the Learning* (Senge, 2006). This process of problem identification is designed to help teams or individuals realize assumptions or generalizations that they make given their data, and to try to remove bias from problem identification. Essentially, when one is on the way "up" the *Ladder of Inference,* the question "why" is asked at every level of problem identification. So, consider using the process with the earlier example of the DNP and her team in a home care professional organization.

> *Problem:* I can't get nurses to use evidence in their home care practice.
> WHY?
> *Problem:* They don't want to come in and learn about evidence-based practice.
> WHY?
> *Problem:* All of the agencies are competing with each other, and they all dislike each other. It's really impacting patient care.
> WHY?
> *Problem:* They are competitors. They want greater market share, they need it for their bottom line. They try to take patients from each other. They try to entice providers to refer to them. It's really a problem.

As you can see, using the *Ladder of Inference* led this team to a very different problem than was originally identified. The team at the professional organization now can work on the problem at hand—the problem that is truly impacting patient care—and a very different set of strategies will need to be developed than strategies that may have included an EBP workshop. Try this process with a variety of problems, and see how the final problem might be very different from the assumptions initially held by the team.

Hypothesis Regarding Causation

Once the team has decided what the real problem is that it is trying to address, a hypothesis regarding causation should be developed using available data. For instance, in the problem identified above, the director of clinical practice and her team have begun to use their available data to hypothesize about the cause of the problem they are trying to address. In using the *Ladder of Inference* and "why?" questioning technique, the team has identified that competition, struggle for market share that affects the organizational bottom line, and recruitment strategies for patients and providers have all led to the nurses in the professional organization not being able to collaborate, learn from one another, and work together toward a common goal. Patient care has been impacted. The team now has a focus for its attention, the actual cause of the problem at hand.

Another method for causal hypothesis generation comes from the quality and safety improvement movement and is known as *root-cause analysis*. Although The Joint Commission has mandated root-cause analysis of sentinel events and errors since 1997 (Agency for Healthcare Research and Quality [AHRQ], n.d.-a, n.d.-b), root-cause analysis techniques can also be valuable to teams that are trying to identify the actual causes of problems they are trying to solve, even prior to a sentinel event occurrence. Typically, root-cause analysis involves following a pre-specified team protocol that begins with data collection and reconstruction or observation of the problem area through a variety of methods, including record review if applicable, direct observation and participation, and participant interviews. The team should then analyze the sequence of events that seems to lead to the problem, with the goals of identifying how the problem occurs and why the problem occurs. Consider the following team problem that has been identified, and the process that the team uses to identify the root cause.

A team of nurses, physicians, and the clinical nursing director for the surgical areas of a tertiary care hospital are faced with the problem of surgical case delays. The problem and its ramifications are clear; surgical case delays lead to patient dissatisfaction and heightened anxiety, provider dissatisfaction, and increased overtime costs as staff must be held past their scheduled shifts to complete the surgical cases. Provider fatigue has the potential to increase surgical errors.

The team undertakes a root-cause analysis. The team first starts with a brainstorming session that identifies all of the systems that are involved or potentially involved in the delays. These include surgical outpatient offices, operating room (OR) scheduling departments, admissions and pre-admission testing units, nursing services, transport services, housekeeping services, surgeons, and surgical staff. The team performs a record review of randomly selected full surgical days, analyzing the start and end time of each surgical case scheduled in each operating room for 7 randomly selected days in 1 month. The team also reviews records of patient arrival times, transport notification times, and room turnover times. Given these data, the team narrows the problem down to two windows of time during which delays seem to be occurring. These time periods include the time between patient arrival in the admissions department and patient arrival in the surgical holding area, and the time between the end of one surgical case and the beginning of the next surgical case in the surgical suites.

The next step for the team is observation of patient flow. Having narrowed down the windows of time where delays are occurring, the team spends time observing the patient admission and transport process, and the process for room turnover. After observation, the team also interviews the managers and staff in each system involved in the delays.

Once all of the data are collected, the team meets to analyze the delays. The root cause of the delays seems to be twofold. Organizational policy dictates that even well adults who come to the admission department to be admitted for a surgical case are required to be transported via wheelchair to the operating room. The transport department has its busiest time of the day in the early morning, when patients are being transported from multiple hospital units for early morning testing. Therefore, the transport department is often delayed in the morning getting patients to the surgical area. This early morning delay leads to a trickle-down effect, causing surgical delays all day as early morning cases are delayed. The second cause is a delay in room turnover. After benchmarking with like institutions, the team finds that the average turnover time for an operating room is 7 minutes. Turnover in this organization is about 23 minutes. Turnover delays are multifaceted; housekeeping services are frequently understaffed during peak OR times, surgical supplies and instrument sterilization are often difficult to find due to space issues in the OR, and staff breaks are strictly scheduled, causing delays as staff may not be available when ORs are ready.

The team has now clearly identified the causes of the problems in this system and can move onto setting their intended outcomes and planning actions to remedy these system problems.

Table 6.3 lists 20 codes frequently used to classify problem causes in a health care environment and can guide the team's thinking about future actions. For instance, if the team classifies the root cause of a problem in the area of knowledge-based behaviors, they will want to attend to educational interventions to increase knowledge in that particular area. Conversely, if the team identifies the root cause of a problem in the category of management priorities, a very different strategy will need to be developed. Teams that work together over time can use these assigned codes for tracking and trending of problem areas, or can use these codes to understand the common threads that drive problems in their organization, and plan to provide attention in those areas. Problems that consistently occur in the area of culture, for instance, would call for organizational attention to issues related to organizational priorities, approaches, and behaviors.

Consider the above example and the use of this classification system for the multifaceted problem causes uncovered during the root-cause analysis. Problems are occurring in the areas of management (staffing levels for transport and housekeeping services at critical time periods), design (unable to find or access key equipment due to lack of storage space), and protocols/procedures and culture (strict policies

TABLE 6.3
The Eindhoven Classification Model for a Medical Domain

CATEGORY	DESCRIPTION	CODE
Latent errors	**Errors that result from underlying system failures**	
Technical	Refers to physical items, such as equipment, physical installations, software, materials, labels, and forms	
External	Technical failures beyond the control and responsibility of the investigating organization	TEX
Design	Failures due to poor design of equipment, software, labels, or forms	TD
Construction	Construction failures despite correct design	TC
Materials	Material defects not classified under TD or TC	TM
Organizational		
External	Failures at an organizational level beyond the control and responsibility of the investigating organization	OEX
Transfer of knowledge	Failures resulting from inadequate measures taken to ensure that situational or domain-specific knowledge or information is transferred to all new or inexperienced staff	OK
Protocols/ procedures	Failures related to the quality and availability of the protocols within the department (too complicated, inaccurate, unrealistic, absent, or poorly presented)	OP
Management priorities	Internal management decisions in which safety is relegated to an inferior position in the face of conflicting demands or objectives; this is a conflict between production needs and safety (e.g., decisions about staffing levels)	OM
Culture	Failures resulting from the collective approach to risk and attendant modes of behavior in the investigating organization	OC
Active errors (human)	**Errors or failures resulting from human behavior**	
External	Human failures originating beyond the control and responsibility of the investigating organization	HEX
Knowledge-based behaviors		
Knowledge-based errors	The inability of an individual to apply existing knowledge to a novel situation	HKK

TABLE 6.3
The Eindhoven Classification Model for a Medical Domain (*continued*)

CATEGORY	DESCRIPTION	CODE
Rule-based behaviors		
Qualification	Incorrect fit between an individual's qualifications, training, or education and a particular tast	HRQ
Coordination	Lack of task coordination within a health care team in an organization	HRC
Verification	Failures in the correct and complete assessment of a situation, including relevant conditions of the patient and materials to be used, before starting the intervention	HRV
Intervention	Failures that result from faulty task planning (selecting the wrong protocol) and/or execution (selecting the right protocol but carrying it out incorrectly)	HRI
Monitoring	Failures during monitoring of the process or patient status during or after the intervention	HRM
Skill-based behaviors		
Slips	Failures in performance of fine motor skills	HSS
Tripping	Failures in whole-body movements	HST
Other		
Patient-related factor	Failures related to patient characteristics or conditions that influence treatment and are beyond staff control	PRF
Unclassifiable	Failures that cannot be classified in any other category	X

Source: Reprinted from Battles, Kaplan, Van der Schaaf, and Shea (1998), with permission from *Archives of Pathology & Laboratory Medicine*. Copyright 1998. College of American Pathologists.

related to patient transport with little flexibility, organizational behaviors around break times). The team can use these classifications to broaden their thinking about the root cause of problems, and develop tailored actions to solve organizational problems.

Teams can make use of online training resources for root-cause analysis such as those found at www.healthinsight.org/Internal/Incident_Investigation-RCA.html to learn more about the root-cause analysis process and tools.

Intended Outcomes

As the team addresses the identified problem and the root cause of the problem it is faced with, it will want to think about the intended outcomes of its work. In the example of the professional organization made up of competing entities, the intended outcome might be collaboration at the level of shared knowledge development for all member nurses. This outcome is an incremental outcome, designed to take a first step toward changing the climate of competition between organizations. This incremental outcome is much different than, and more realistic than, trying to solve the problem of competition among organizations. In some cases, like the surgical example presented earlier, the intended outcome is based on a benchmark. So, if the national average for surgical room turnover in like organizations in the United States is 7 minutes, the team can set an intended outcome with this in mind. They may set incremental outcomes, like decreasing the turnover time by half in the first 6 months, and decreasing to the national average in 1 year. The choice belongs to the team and the organization, and depends upon the available resources, personnel, and what is realistic given the multiple influences affecting the problem.

Objectives

Once the team has decided on an intended outcome, it can begin to set objectives for its work together. What is an objective for a team project? An objective is a clear and measurable statement related to the work of the team. The objective or objectives will be specific in relation to intent, timing, budget, and other areas of importance to the project. An example of a strong objective for the surgical problem detailed earlier might be:

> By June 30, the team will develop and implement, in collaboration with the department of transport, an alternative staffing plan that will allow for the availability of six dedicated full-time equivalents of transport professionals during the hours of 7 a.m. and 10 a.m. each weekday for patient transport from the admitting department to the surgical department.

In evaluating this objective, is it clear? Measurable? Specific with regard to time and numbers? And finally, will each team member understand what he or she is trying to accomplish? The answer is yes to all of these questions for this objective. This is the type of strong objective the team should work toward.

Mathis (2011) has developed the **DISCO** method for teams to consider as a process when trying to set measurable project objectives. These include:

D: Detail Specifics: Mathis (2011) believes that teams should provide as much information as possible in their objectives and that the objectives should be very specific. The team should know exactly what work is required through the detail that is provided in the objectives.

I: Include Qualitative and Quantitative Measurements: Nurses and other health care providers are familiar with the development of measurable goals in everyday patient care. However, how can the team be sure that project objectives are measurable? Mathis (2011) suggests that the team asks the question "Can we measure this?" with each objective it develops. Qualitative measures that may be used by a health care team may include results of interviews, focus groups, or sometimes satisfaction measures. Quantitative measures are based on numbers. The team may include objectives that can be measured in terms of time, budget, incidents or occurrences, or benchmarks.

S: Seek Consensus With the Team: Seeking consensus from the beginning of the team's work together related to its objectives helps to keep everyone on the team moving in the same direction. When teams understand and agree upon objectives, they are more likely to work together to achieve those objectives.

C: Create a Reasonable Approach in Obtaining Those Objectives: The approach will be discussed in more detail later in our Strategies section, but in the planning phase, the key point is to be sure that the approach is understood by all team members, decreasing conflict in the implementation process.

O: Operate in a Methodical Time Frame: Mathis (2011) advocates for setting up a time frame and following it. The team may use some of its teamwork strategies to be sure that it is following its timelines. Meeting software may be used to track timelines. Daily scrums might use timelines as a daily touchpoint for progress. Team agendas may include the project timeline for each team meeting. Team time should be spent focusing on the timeline and whether it is realistic and being met by the team's work.

Strategies: Strategies are actions that will be taken by the team to meet the objectives. Strategies should also be specific and be developed by consensus. Frequently, strategies will involve many systems outside of the team. Strategies for engagement of those systems should be arrived at by the team. Strategies are also where team strengths can be used. In the surgical example above, recall the objective:

> By June 30, the team will develop and implement, in collaboration with the department of transport, an alternative staffing plan that will allow for the availability of six dedicated FTE's of transport professionals during the hours of 7 a.m. and 10 a.m. each weekday for patient transport from the admitting department to the surgical department.

What strategies can be developed by the team to meet this objective? First, the team needs to consider what other systems are involved in this objective. Their list might include the organizational administration, transport department, the finance department, the admissions department, and the surgical department. The team should first develop a strategy for engagement of these systems. They may decide to prioritize engagement. So they may develop an initial strategy to engage with the transport departmental administration to develop the plan. Once the plan is developed, they may develop a strategy to engage the finance department to analyze the cost of the plan. They may also ask the finance department to work with the surgical department to analyze the cost of the delays and the cost offsets for development of this plan if surgical delays are decreased. Alternatively, the team may decide to develop a strategy to engage every department in the planning. Decisions like these will depend on the team's knowledge of the organizational culture, structure, climate, and the strengths of the team members.

The Ladder of Inference discussed earlier can also be used by team members for action planning. If you recall, in problem clarification, the team asked the question "why?" as they moved up the Ladder of Inference. Once they reach the top of the Ladder of Inference and are ready to plan action, they might use the question "how?" in a similar manner to identify their clear strategies. So, in the objective above, the team is going to develop an alternative plan for staffing of the transport service. Below, the use of the "how?" question allows them to develop clear strategies for implementation.

> *Action:* Develop an alternative plan for transport department staffing for surgical patients.

HOW?

Action: Engage the transport department administration in the work of the team.

HOW?

Action: The team leader will meet with the transport department administration to present the results of the root-cause analysis demonstrating that delays in transport of surgical patients from the admission department are leading to progressive surgical delays throughout the day.

HOW?

Action: The team leader will contact the transport administrator and invite him to meet within the next week.

This process of asking "how" allows the team to get to a clear strategy for action to meet its objective. Regardless of the strategies developed, strategies should be clear, related to meeting the objectives, and agreed upon by the team from the outset.

Resources Required

Teams will want to carefully consider the resources that will be required in order to implement the strategies they are developing. A broad array of resources should be considered. Resources for team projects will typically fall into two categories: person resources and nonperson resources. Person resources include the knowledge, skills, and strengths of team members. Also included is the time that people will need to spend on the project, and perhaps an accounting of how that time will take them away from other activities. Also included are any person resources needed to implement the plan. Nonperson resources include equipment, space, facilities, and supplies. The team may want to develop a chart like Tables 6.4 and 6.5 to help them identify the resources needed to implement their strategies.

Action Steps

Action steps are those actual activities that must be planned in order to carry out the strategies developed by the team. Depending upon your team's working style, culture, and ground rules, action steps may be very specific and delineated at each meeting. The action steps bring logic to the process of project planning. To begin planning actions,

TABLE 6.4
Project Planning Resource Analysis: Person Resources

STRATEGY	SKILLS NEEDED	NAME OF TEAM MEMBER	SKILLS LEVEL	START DATE	END DATE	COST

Source: Adapted from Singh (n.d.).

TABLE 6.5
Project Planning Resource Analysis: Nonperson Resources

STRATEGY	RESOURCE NEEDED	TIME NEEDED	DATE OR DATES NEEDED

Source: Adapted from Singh (n.d.).

team members can brainstorm all the possible steps that are required to complete. Next, the team will want to prioritize these actions. Team members will want to come to consensus on priorities for actions, asking which are most important, which are time sensitive, or which must be completed prior to other actions. The team's goal should be to develop a logical list of steps for the team to follow. In creating the action steps, the team will also want to set some timelines. They should consider realistic time frames for accomplishing actions and what time periods are critical for taking action as the team moves forward with its plan. Finally, the team will want to build some accountability mechanisms into the action steps. Using their ground rules, teams can decide on the accountability system that is most appropriate to their work together. These may include reports to the group or an individual, most likely the team leader, who is charged with checking in with team members to make sure that actions are proceeding as planned. Project planning and implementation software, which will be described later, can be used to document the completion of actions.

Evaluation

Typically, project evaluation includes three components: *process, outcomes, and impact*. If the team has gone through this systematic process of project planning, process and outcome evaluation of the project will be easy. Evaluation of process involves looking at what is being done and can occur during the project to allow for improvement. Process evaluation should emerge easily from the project strategies, and action steps if they have been developed with specificity, are time limited, and are measurable. In the first step of the project plan, the team set a specific intended outcome, which will be the grand measure of the success of the project. If that outcome is specific and measurable, the team should have no difficulty measuring the success in reaching that outcome. Finally, impact evaluation considers the longer-term results of the project, including the unintentional consequences of the project, long-term costs, and the acceptability of the change over time in the organization. In their evaluation handbook, the Joint Information Systems Committee (JISC) of the United Kingdom suggests that a team can use certain questions that will help to focus the type of evaluation that is needed. Table 6.6 outlines some of those questions as they might relate to a health care project evaluation plan.

Regardless of the type of evaluation chosen, there are some key considerations related to evaluation that the team must agree upon in its planning. These include timing, factors to evaluate, questions to address in the evaluation, methods and sources of data, and measures of success (Glenaffric, 2007).

Timing

Teams will consider the appropriate timing for evaluation to occur. Process evaluation may be ongoing throughout the project, and can in fact help to improve outcomes, as processes can be adjusted as the project moves forward based upon the knowledge gained. Outcome evaluation may also be ongoing, as short-, intermediate-, and long-term outcomes may be set by the project team, and will need to be evaluated at the appropriate time in the project. Finally, impact evaluation will likely be done after the project has been completed, and will allow the team to look at the lasting effects of the change. Some key questions face the team in decisions about the timing of their evaluation, depending on the type of evaluation and the intervening factors in the project plan implementation. For instance, when will effects be expected? When will data be available? How long do we expect effects to last? When will effects be fully realized? In a project like the surgical project detailed in this chapter, the team will likely take months planning the project. Process evaluation may be planned according to the steps they have outlined for action. Perhaps the change, once approved, will be implemented incrementally, affecting when the full impact of the intervention will be seen in the system. Data about turnover times in ORs

TABLE 6.6
Evaluation Type and Suggested Questions for Project Evaluation

EVALUATION TYPE	SUGGESTED QUESTIONS
Process	Does the process that was developed work for team members? Others?
	Is the team satisfied with the process?
	Are actions helping to meet objectives?
	Are there any ethical/legal/quality/safety issues emerging?
	Are resources being used appropriately?
	What are the barriers or facilitators?
	Who else needs to be involved?
	What skills are we calling upon frequently?
	What skills are we missing?
	What are the next steps?
Outcome	What is the desired change?
	Is the change occurring?
	Are the changes effective in meeting the overall outcome?
	To what extent is the desired change occurring?
Impact	What are the unintended outcomes of the change?
	To what extent have the desired benefits been achieved?
	To what extent have they been sustained?
	What are the costs? Benefits?
	Is the change cost-effective?

Source: Adapted from Glenaffric Ltd (2007).

might not be available until medical record reviews are completed. All of these will impact when this team plans to perform an outcome evaluation. In the example of the team that is implementing an intervention to facilitate collaboration among home care nurses, timing is even more crucial. After an education intervention, how long does it take to realize real change? How long do we expect the effects of that intervention to last? Again, these questions are crucial for the team to consider in their deliberations relative to the timing of evaluation.

Factors to Evaluate

The team must consider what factors it will evaluate. Objectives may have multiple parts that the team can consider in its evaluation. So, in the surgical case example, the team might decide to evaluate whether it met its time deadline. The team may decide to evaluate whether key stakeholders were involved in the project. It may also opt to evaluate whether the recommendation for six FTEs during the specified times of the day was implemented. Each of these provides the team with a different piece of information, all relating to the evaluation of the overall intended outcome. If key stakeholders were not involved, or if the full recommendation was not implemented, then the team may not see the reduction in OR turnover time at the level anticipated. Considering carefully which aspects of each objective can have an impact on the overall intended outcomes for the project will help the team get a good picture of what factors led to success or failure.

Questions to Address

The team will want to consider what questions it wants to address in its evaluation. This discussion will allow the team to really decide what members want to know about the success of their project. Glenaffric (2007) suggests that the five Es can help a team think about what it wants to know in its evaluation. The five Es along with some health care project planning questions the team might ask include:

- *Efficacy:* Does the plan work? Does it work like it was intended to work?
- *Efficiency:* Does the plan use resources responsibly?
- *Elegance:* Is the plan "pleasing" to those who are working within the system?
- *Effectiveness:* Does it attain the intended outcome?
- *Ethicality:* Is the plan moral? Ethical? Safe?

Methods and Sources of Data

The team will want to consider the methods that it will use for evaluation, as well as the sources of data that will be available for the evaluation. A variety of methods are available for undertaking an evaluation, including chart review, records review, questionnaires, surveys, observation, focus groups, interviews, and others. Considerations for team members in selecting a method include skill of the team with the method, supports for the particular method, time, expense, and availability. Chart reviews and record reviews may be time-consuming, but the data are generally available, and the method is low cost. However, the team may want to measure an indicator that is not available in these data, like user satisfaction or perceived collaboration among providers. The team may want to consider a questionnaire or survey for collecting data for these types of indicators. Skills in questionnaire or survey development, sample selection, and analysis will be important for the team to collect valid and reliable data using these methods. Observation, focus groups or interviews may allow a team to perform a more in-depth evaluation of processes, acceptability, and perceptions of barriers and facilitators, but are more time-consuming and costly forms of evaluation for the team. The team needs to consider the best method to provide them with the data needed to evaluate their program.

Measures of Success

The team will want to select the indicators of their success. These indicators will provide evidence that the team was successful in achieving change. Indicators of change typically evaluate change from a baseline, so it will be important to establish a baseline indicator against which to measure progress. In the surgical case example, the team knows that the baseline for OR turnover in their organization is 23 minutes. This baseline forms the basis for their measure of success. An indicator of success will be a reduction in turnover time from the organizational baseline.

TOOLS FOR PROJECT PLANNING

Teams can make use of multiple project planning tools available through a variety of resources. The most popular project planning tool used in health care planning is the Logic Model developed by the Kellogg Foundation and available free for download from their website (www.wkkf.org/knowledge-center/resources/2006/02/WK-Kellogg-Foundation-Logic-Model-Development-Guide.aspx). The Kellogg Foundation Logic Model was designed as a visual tool to allow program planners to consider all of the components of project planning outlined earlier in this chapter.

A logic model is "a systematic and visual way to present and share your understanding of the relationships among the resources you have to operate your program, the activities you plan, and the changes or results you hope to achieve" (WK Kellogg Foundation, 2004, p. 1). A logic model allows the team to develop a picture of how it envisions the program to work, and what it will take in order to make the project

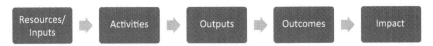

FIGURE 6.3 The basic logic model.

Source: Reprinted and adapted with permission from WK Kellogg Foundation (2004).

work. The basic logic model components are broken down into two categories—your planned work and your intended results. Figure 6.3 illustrates the basic logic model.

Your Planned Work

This section of a logic model demonstrates what resources the team will need to implement the project and also what the team intends to actually do during the project period. The two sections of the logic model that fall under this category are *resources* and *program activities*. *Resources* are those things that are available to the team in order to do the work of the project, and are sometimes called *inputs*. *Resources* can include human, financial, organizational, community, information technology, and infrastructure that will be able to be directed toward the work. By delineating the resources available and needed, the team can identify gaps in resources and will be able to develop a plan for filling those gaps. *Program activities* include what the team will do with the resources available. Program activities are the "processes, tools, events, technology and actions that are an intentional part of the program implementation" (WK Kellogg, 2004, p. 2). All of these activities are directed toward bringing about the intended results.

Your Intended Results

This section of the logic model helps the team delineate all of the project's intended outcomes. Included in this section of the logic model are *outputs, outcomes,* and *impact*. Outputs are the products of program activities. These might include "types, levels and targets" of services to be provided by the project. *Outcomes* are as expected the specific changes that are expected to be seen as a result of the project. Short-term and long-term outcomes are included. Finally, *impact* is the realization of the change at the organizational level that will be realized over the long term because of the changes introduced by the project.

TABLE 6.7
Logic Model: Surgical Delay Project Team

YOUR PLANNED WORK			YOUR INTENDED RESULTS	
Resources/ Inputs →	Activities →	Outputs →	Outcomes →	Impact
Data	Review OR records Review charts Observe surgical patient flow from admission to arrival in suite	Number of surgical patients in OR on time per day Number of surgeries per day	OR turnover time decreased to 12 minutes within first 6 months OR turnover time decreased to 7 minutes within first year	Increased staff and patient satisfaction Increased surgical volume Decreased surgical errors due to staff fatigue
Buy in of all impacted departments	Observe OR turnover process Engage impacted departments in discussion of solution Include admissions, transport, finance, surgical departments	Number of overtime shifts needed per week due to late cases Number of surgical errors attributed to provider fatigue		
Funding for implementation	Develop plan to increase transport service availability during peak OR times Evaluate cost of plan and potential cost savings Present plan to key stakeholders Implement and evaluate plan to increase transport services			

A sample logic model for the surgical problem presented earlier in this chapter is found in Table 6.7.

MANAGING CHANGE

Most teams are working together to influence change. It has been said that no one likes change except a wet baby. However, anyone who has ever changed a wet baby knows that oftentimes babies do not like change either! So, how does an effective team manage change?

Most change efforts fail due to lack of planning. Again, just like with setting up the team and carefully planning the project, taking the time to plan change will allow the team to realize its preferred outcomes more often, and in less time than with unplanned efforts. Teams managing change must consider the people, priorities, business, communication, and resistance in their planning. Although many classic change theories exist, most have these elements in common.

People

Change involves two sets of people: those who are driving the change to occur and those who are impacted by the change. Although in many organizational structures those who are driving the change are at the top of the organization, as organizations flatten, and employees and teams are empowered to facilitate change in an organization, this traditional view of top-down change is being challenged. Regardless of whether change is top-down or bottom-up, the two groups, those who drive the change and those who are impacted by the change, must be considered by the team in all of their activities.

Managing the drivers of change may challenge a team in a number of ways. A driver of change may be the sponsor of the team, and therefore may have some control over the team, or the team may be responsible to that sponsor for their outcomes. In fact, the team may be in existence because of the sponsor's need to drive change, so the team's very existence can be dependent upon that driver of change. Drivers of change typically want change to happen quickly, and the team may be challenged to convince the driver of change that a deliberate, planned process should be undertaken. The team needs to be responsive to the needs of the driver of change, but also must balance this responsiveness with planning. Because poor planning in change efforts may lead to project delays, increased costs, and eventual failure, the team should make the business case to the driver of change regarding the need for deliberate planning. The team should be pre-pared to answer common questions by drivers of change, answers that have been derived from team discussion, work, and delibera-tion. Some common questions that drivers of change may challenge a team with include:

- When can the change be completed?
- What is the required investment by our organization in human and other capital?
- How will this change impact our clinical performance? In financial performance?
- What is the return on this investment to be realized with this change in 1 year, 5 years?
- How much improvement in clinical care will be realized? In finan-cial performance?
- What are the potential unintended outcomes of this change?

The team should include these questions as part of their project plan-ning for any change. Later in this chapter, we will discuss some com-mon project planning techniques that teams can use to answer some of these questions.

Managing those people who the change affects is also a challenge for teams. Lack of management of change for this group can result in resistance, discontent, decreased productivity and a higher turnover rate among employees, or a loss of patients in a system. In clinical care, these can impact patient care, lead to an unsafe clinical care environment, or impact the numbers and types of services that an organization can provide. Unlike change drivers, people involved in change at this level have one question—"how will this change affect me and my work or my care?" These are the people who are most likely involved in the day-to-day operations of the organization, or those who are receiving care in the area where change is being con-templated. These are employees, volunteers, patients, and families, who may lack the big picture of operations in the organization, and are focused on how a change might affect their ability to provide or receive excellent care. Patients and families may be concerned with how a change might impact the care that they are used to receiv-ing and expect from a particular organization. The concerns of those impacted by change are deeply personal, and require careful work by the team to allow for successful implementation of the change. So, the team must be prepared to answer the following set of questions for this group:

- How will this impact my day-to-day job?
- How will this change impact the care that I provide?
- Will this change impact the systems that I depend upon to provide excellent care?
- How will this change impact the care that I or my family receives in this organization?
- Are there alternate methods of change that can minimize the change on me and my work?

The bottom line in considering the people side of change is considering all stakeholders, respecting all perspectives, and planning to minimize the resistance to change from all people involved.

Priorities

In planning change, the team must carefully examine priorities for change from a variety of perspectives. What is the organizational priority being addressed? Teams should go back to the organization's strategic plan and see how the planned change is linked back to the bigger organizational picture. So, for example, if the team is planning a change that involves development of a system for performance evaluation at all levels of the organization, they may link that change to an organizational goal that says "invest in our people to retain the best and brightest." A team considering the development of a new service line to provide transitional care services by advanced practice nurses to decrease re-hospitalizations in frail elders can link their planning for change to a strategic goal that states "grow existing services and identify new opportunities to meet the health care needs of the state and region" and another that states "provide safe, quality, patient-centered care to every patient." Finally, with the advent of decreased payment for re-hospitalizations from some payers, the team might also link this initiative to the organizational goal "develop a sustainable operational plan through innovative programs." Linking back to organizational priorities is not only strategic but will also help the team demonstrate to multiple stakeholders how their work "fits" with the organization.

What other priorities might the team consider in their planning? The priorities of the team sponsor will certainly be taken into account. The team will want to spend time at the beginning of its work to clarify the priorities of the sponsor. In the case of the team developing a performance evaluation system for all levels of employees, what is the priority for the sponsor? Ease of use? Applicability across multiple classifications of workers? Cost to implement? Recognition of excellence? Retention of employees? Removing weak employees? As this short list demonstrates, strategies for planning change can be impacted immensely by the priorities of the "owner" of the work. A system that is developed for low cost may not be able to be applicable across multiple classifications of workers. Likewise, designing a program to recognize excellence may be different than one that is merely designed to retain employees. The team should be clear from the outset about the priorities of those who own the change.

The priorities of the people impacted by the change should also be taken into consideration. In the case of developing a transitional care program for frail elders that is implemented by advanced practice nurses (APNs), the team will want to consider not only the priorities of the organization but also those of the APN, those of patients and families, and those of their primary care providers. Although the APN might have as a priority the ability to function to the full scope of practice, the primary care provider may have as a priority to maintain this frail elder as a patient, and may be threatened by the introduction of another caregiver. The priority of families and caregivers might be to keep their elder family member safe, and may consider the hospital or the emergency room the safest environment, rather than the home. Competing priorities will need to be considered and carefully thought through as a change strategy is being developed.

Business

When planning change, the team will also want to consider the business side of change for an organization. Although teams may not be experts in the business part of the equation, the team can reach out to experts who can help them think through and develop the business case for a change. However, many of the business considerations are within the expertise of a team. In addition to questions reviewed earlier, like financial impact and return on investment, the team will want to think through issues such as competition in the market place, market share, regulatory barriers to the proposed change, and possible innovative funding mechanisms or opportunities to support the change. For example, suppose a team in long-term care is considering the introduction of "medication aides" to be supervised by the registered nurse in a long-term care agency. Questions for consideration include:

- What is happening in the marketplace of long-term care?
- Have other organizations implemented this system? What has the financial impact been?
- Will a program such as this impact our market share by increasing the satisfaction of our residents and their families? If so, how?
- Are there regulatory barriers to this change, such as rules that forbid the delegation of medication administration by the registered nurse? If so, what will it take to change these rules?
- Are there safety issues that could impact our bottom line and our quality of care? How do we overcome those safety concerns?
- Are there potential opportunities for funding demonstration projects to evaluate this change?

Reviewing these types of questions does not require a full team of business people, but rather a team dedicated to look at potential change from a variety of perspectives, and to be prepared to answer these types of questions when asked.

Communication

In planning for change by preparing for the questions we have reviewed thus far, the team will also want to plan for how it will communicate the change. As discussed in Chapter 5, a communication plan should be considered that extends from the beginning of the team's work together until the planned change has been evaluated. What needs to be considered in a communication plan?

First, the team needs to know that as soon as their members are appointed, others are aware that "something is going on." Who will communicate on behalf of the team? Is there a designated team spokesperson? Are all team members empowered to speak on behalf of the team? The team will want to carefully consider, along with the sponsor, what they will communicate with others. What will they tell those who ask about why they exist? What they are planning? Why they were chosen? Carefully considering answers to these questions may impact later acceptance of the change. Likewise, having the team provide consistent answers to questions such as these may help to minimize resistance and decrease speculation about the team's work. Teams will also want to consider when they will communicate with others about their work. Some teams choose to release an immediate statement about their existence and purpose, with a promise of later details as work progresses. Teams might ask to be placed regularly on the agenda of key committees to provide updates on their work. Another opportunity to communicate might be quarterly newsletters, regular e-mail communications, or social media sites. One recent team that was working on the renovation of a clinical simulation laboratory provided weekly Facebook updates regarding plans, inviting feedback at each step of planning. Another team involved in the development of a strategic plan placed the results of its work each month in a blog and invited participation via the blog or in public forums held throughout the planning process. Some teams choose to strategically include small groups in their communication from the outset of their work, with the groups they communicate with becoming larger and larger as the change is planned, implemented, and evaluated. Regardless of how the team plans to communicate, the bottom line is there should be as comprehensive a plan for communication of change as there is for the change itself. This planning can help to allay fears, answer questions, and eventually increase buy-in by the stakeholders of the change.

Resistance

Even with great planning, it is rare for a change to be met without resistance from someone or some group. Resistance can be due to a variety of factors, including perceived threat, impact on relationships, feeling coerced, lack of knowledge, poor communication, and an unclear cost–benefit ratio for stakeholders.

> *Perceived threat:* It is human nature to be cautious about the unknown. We all feel uncomfortable and sometimes threatened when we are entering an uncertain environment. People in an organization may feel that a change threatens their ability to do their job. Others may feel that a change might cause them to lose their job. Still others feel threatened just by the loss of the status quo.
>
> *Impact on relationships:* As social beings, we are all involved in relationships with others in our organization. Whether they are reporting relationships, peer relationships, mentoring relationships, or partnerships to achieve outcomes, most people gain stability in their work from those relationships. Change that impacts those relationships makes people uncomfortable and may lead to resistance to change.

Feeling coerced: We all like to feel in control of our own lives, whether at work or in our personal spheres. But oftentimes, in the face of change in organizations, people feel that they have no choice but to go along with the change, however it impacts them. Although we are not necessarily resistant to change, we are resistant to feeling out of control of that change.

Lack of knowledge: Lack of knowledge is a key factor in resistance to change. Having incomplete or incorrect information can lead to strong resistance to change. Rumors have a way of following any change, and they can provide people with incorrect information upon which to base their opinions of change.

Poor communication: Poor communication is a key contributor to resistance to change. Communication that is ambiguous, conflicting, or untimely endangers the success of the change through feeding resistance. Poor communication can introduce chaos into the change process.

Unclear cost–benefit ratio: Change takes work. A lack of understanding of the payoff for that work is a key component in resistance to change. Remember that individuals affected by change are primarily interested in the impact of the change on them or their job. If those people cannot see that the work that change takes will have a benefit to them in the improvement of some aspect of their work or life, they are more likely to resist that change.

How does the team use all of these considerations about resistance to change in their planning? First, realizing the multiple reasons for resistance is essential. Considering the potential areas of resistance and the possible resistors (either individuals or groups) should be a key activity in any team's planning of change. For example, if a team of nurse and health care administrators is planning a building project that will open a new tower at a tertiary hospital, what are the areas of potential resistance? Cost is an obvious one. But what about other hospitals in the area and their concerns about market share? How about regulatory bodies that are concerned about the need for this expansion of services? And, what about the patient population that asks how their care will be disrupted during this 2-year building project? Potential resistance in this case is both internal and external. After identifying these areas of potential resistance, the team can consider them in their planning. Bergman (2009) suggests three steps to deal with resistance to change that may feel somewhat uncomfortable to teams at first, but can be built into team planning:

1. Define the outcome you want.
2. Suggest a path to achieve it.
3. Allow people to reject your path as long as they choose an alternate route to the same destination.

This method allows people to decrease uncertainty and feelings of threat about the future, and allows them to have some control while achieving the outcome that is desired by the team. Coupled with good communication, and the provision of information that is clear and easy to understand, this strategy might be the key to a team's successful plan to overcome resistance.

SUMMARY AND NEXT STEPS

Forming a team is only the first step in the process of team success. Working together is where the rubber meets the road in team processes. Careful planning allows all team members and partners to have input into the team's strategies, and will pay off in the long term by decreasing implementation problems. The tools in this chapter can help teams structure their work, including team meetings, planning approaches to team challenges, using existing tools for project or program planning, and managing change. In the next chapter, methods to measure the success of a team's work together will be discussed.

QUESTIONS FOR THOUGHT

1. Consider the structure of your current team meetings. How might you use the tools presented in this chapter to improve the effectiveness of team meetings?
2. How might technology be used to better communicate the results of team meetings in your organization? How might use of technology improve team communication and transparency?
3. Analyze the steps needed to plan for an upcoming project in your organization. Have all of the steps identified in this chapter, including problem identification, hypothesis generation, intended outcomes, objectives, strategies, resources, action steps, and evaluation plans, been considered? How might you as a team leader influence the planning of this project?
4. Use the DISCO (Mathis, 2011) method to develop measurable project objectives for your team's next project. How might using this method improve the work of your team?

5. Using the measurable project objectives you have developed, design a prospective evaluation plan for your team's next project. How can you include an evaluation of process, outcome, and impact in your evaluation design?

6. Develop a logic model for a real or potential project for your organization. What parts of the logic model seem most important to your project's success? The development of which components challenge your team the most?

7. Describe how change normally occurs in your organization. How could you design a change using the methods described in this chapter that would improve on current change methods?

SEVEN

Measuring Team and Partnership Success in Nursing and Health Care Environments

I am easily satisfied with the very best.
                    —Winston Churchill

LEARNING OBJECTIVES

1. Define the elements of team success.
2. Identify key questions for team self-evaluation.
3. Analyze the advantages and disadvantages of external evaluation of team success.
4. Describe the use of standardized methods for team evaluation.

*H*ow do we know when a team is successful? Is a team successful if they win games? Influence positive change? Function smoothly? Fail to accomplish their goals but work well together? Measurement of team success is a multifaceted undertaking and depends on how team success has been defined. For some teams, the outcome or end product of their work together is their measure of success. For others, even if they do not meet their goals, working together cohesively is a measure of success for them and their organization, and may have future implications for the organization. This chapter will provide teams with tools to measure their performance as a team, and to evaluate the outcomes of their work together as a team.

151

DEFINING TEAM SUCCESS

Eickenberry (2007) has suggested that team success is dependent on seven elements found in all high-performing teams. These elements should not be a surprise to readers of this book, and include:

- *Commitment:* Highly successful teams are committed to their work. They share vision, have a keen understanding of their m ission, and are committed to making the team work.
- *Trust:* Not only are team members committed to a common cause, but they have also built trust in each other and in the team's processes. This trust allows them to freely express ideas, and to solve conflicts with respect.
- *Purpose:* The highly effective team understands their purpose and how it links back to the organization's mission and goals. They understand that their purpose transcends the work of the team and can impact the entire organization.
- *Communication:* The successful team has developed methods for clear communication between team members, with the organization, and outside of the organization.
- *Involvement:* In an effective team, all members have a role. Building on their strengths, each team member understands what they bring to the table for the team. They also understand the roles of others and value their strengths as well. Involvement at all levels of a team's development and work is a priority for all team members.
- *Process orientation:* All highly successful teams have a process orientation for their work. They make use of a variety of tools to assess their strengths, their environment, and organization, and to guide their work.
- *Continuous improvement:* In a successful team, members are constantly learning through their work together. They are learning from each other, and using that knowledge to enhance the team. They are learning from their successes and their failures, purposefully studying each to improve their work.

Consider how this list relates back to the processes of team development that we have discussed throughout this book. For instance, how do these relate to the team charter experience? To team development models? To team meetings? If the time has been taken to purposefully develop the team using the tools presented in this text, the elements for team success should be present.

The challenge, however, for teams is to objectively measure their success as a team. The measurement of team success can be accomplished in a variety of ways. Self-evaluation can be undertaken by the team and its members. External evaluation by managers, sponsors, and peers can also be valuable in measuring teamwork. Finally, objective, standardized measures of team functioning can be used to measure teamwork.

TEAM SELF-EVALUATION

Team self-evaluation has some distinct advantages. First and foremost, no one knows better about the team's work together than the team members themselves. Team members have lived the experience of developing and working as a team and therefore should be in the best position to evaluate their functioning. Unlike outsiders looking at the team, the team understands the structures they have introduced to facilitate their work, and the environment they have created in which to accomplish their goals. The team can look closely at those structures and their environment to evaluate their work together.

If the team has paid attention to the elements of team development outlined in the previous chapters of this book, a framework for self-evaluation is evident. Some potential questions for the team to reflect upon during self-evaluation are found in Table 7.1.

The insights gained by a team during a self-evaluation exercise can be tremendously valuable to its future success. Taking the time to stop and be introspective about how the team functions together is essential. Therefore, team performance self-evaluation should be undertaken at various points in the team's work together. For instance, a team may decide to undertake evaluation after a specific period of time in its work together—at the 6-month or 1-year mark. Or, a team may use externally imposed time periods for self-evaluation, for example, around the time of an organization-wide performance evaluation period. Evidence of team performance and individual contribution to that performance can enhance an individual's performance evaluation immensely. All health care environments today should care about team performance, and inclusion of some sort of evaluative criteria about performance on a team in individual performance appraisals is common. Finally, a team should always take the time to evaluate its work together at the end of the work—not only to evaluate its own success but also to be able to carry forward the successful lessons learned in the team environment to future teams they lead in the organization.

TABLE 7.1
Team Self-Evaluation Guide

TEAM EVALUATION ELEMENTS	POTENTIAL QUESTIONS FOR TEAM SELF-EVALUATION
Strengths and Skills	Have we identified team talents, knowledge, and skills? Have we identified skill gaps? Have we planned our work to optimize team talents and skills? Have we filled skill gaps? How?
Professionalism ■ Honesty and integrity ■ Reliability and responsibility ■ Respect for others ■ Compassion and empathy ■ Self-improvement ■ Self-awareness and knowledge of limits ■ Advocacy ■ Communication and collaboration	Have we committed to the tenets of professionalism? What are some examples of how we have demonstrated that commitment to professionalism? How have we supported each other in developing a professional environment for our work? How have we demonstrated leadership in facilitating a professional environment?

Relational Coordination
■ Communication
  ■ Frequency
  ■ Timeliness
  ■ Accuracy
■ Relationships
  ■ Shared goals
  ■ Shared knowledge
  ■ Mutual respect
	Have we committed to the tenets of relational coordination?
	What are some examples of how we have committed to relational coordination?
	What communication systems have we developed that facilitate frequent, timely, and accurate communication among our team members? With outside stakeholders?
	Have we spent time developing shared goals?
	Are we using a team charter to guide our work together?
	Do we use our team mission and vision to guide our work?
	Are we taking opportunities to share knowledge frequently?
	Are we demonstrating mutual respect through adherence to our agreed-upon ground rules?

(continued)

TABLE 7.1
Team Self-Evaluation Guide (*continued*)

TEAM EVALUATION ELEMENTS	POTENTIAL QUESTIONS FOR TEAM SELF-EVALUATION
Team Transparency	Have we developed an environment that facilitates team transparency? What are the examples of how we have developed a transparent environment? How much do we know about each other's work? How have we intentionally built systems in our work to influence transparency?
Team Development Stage ■ Forming ■ Storming ■ Norming ■ Performing	At what stage of team development are we currently working? How have we developed an environment to facilitate our team development? What are some examples of how we have facilitated that environment? What are our plans to move to a higher level of development? Have we considered the life span of our team—should we be moving to the adjourning phase or should we continue to perform as a team?
Organizational Interface ■ Organizational culture ■ Organizational structure ■ Organizational image ■ Organizational politics ■ Organizational leadership ■ Organizational communication	Have we used our knowledge of the organization to plan and implement our work? What are examples of how we have used our analysis of the organization to facilitate our success as a team? Have we experienced any limitations to our work attributed to elements of organizational culture, structure, image, politics, leadership, communication?

There are certainly some limitations to team self-evaluation. First, self-evaluation is time-consuming. However, the lessons learned from team self-evaluation are invaluable for future work, so the time should be taken for self-evaluation. Next, self-evaluation requires motivation of the team to be introspective. Finally, by its very nature, self-evaluation is subjective. We are not always the best judges of our own performance. However, if the team has worked hard together to develop an environment of communication, sharing, and mutual respect, the subjectivity involved in self-evaluation decreases.

Teams may question with whom in the organization to share the team self-evaluation. The answer to this question will be different for every team, and may be different at different times in the team's development. Periodic team evaluation may simply be shared with the team for its own growth and planning, or perhaps to right its course if the functioning of the team has been evaluated to have moved away from its original plans. At other times, team self-evaluation may be shared with team sponsors. Team sponsors are interested in facilitating the work of the team, and sharing team self-evaluation with the sponsor may have some valuable results for the team's future development. For instance, the sponsor may identify resources that the team can access to improve particular areas of performance. The sponsor may be able to mentor team members in specific skills. The sponsor may also be able to promote the team's strengths through sharing self-evaluation elements in the broader organization. Finally, the team may share the self-evaluation with managers, administrators, and other leaders in the organization. These groups are not only interested in facilitating the work of the team but are also invested in the success of the team and what their success means for organizational outcomes. So, sharing the self-evaluation with those in the organization invested in the team's success may result in the investment in additional resources and attention to the work of the team. Certainly at the end of the team's work together, organizational leaders should be interested in hearing the teamwork lessons learned through the work of the team, and will want to be sure those lessons are shared with future teams throughout the organization.

EXTERNAL EVALUATION OF TEAM SUCCESS

External evaluation of team success has some distinct advantages over self-evaluation. The subjectivity that is involved in self-evaluation may be diminished with external evaluation. Because external evaluators are not as close to the work of the team, they may be able to see some of the strengths and weaknesses of the team's functioning together that team members may not be cognizant of in their work. External evaluators, because they may not have personal relationships with the team members, may be able to be more candid in their observations of the team's work together. However, external evaluation is not without limitations. The advantage of having an insider's view of how the team has set up structures and systems to facilitate its work together is lost with external evaluation. And, if the external evaluator has only a "point in time" evaluation perspective, he or she will not have insights into the history of the trajectory of the team's development over time, the intentionality that went into selection of team members, the skill development that was undertaken during the team's history together, or the team's attention to the development of an environment to facilitate its work. External evaluation, because it is usually not done longitudinally, may only capture a view of the team in its current state, and not the full picture of the team's development that led to its current state.

The selection of external evaluators should be carefully thought out by teams. Attention to the purpose of the evaluation, the intended users of the evaluation, and the knowledge of the external evaluators of the work of the team and of teamwork elements in general should be considered by the team as they consider who they will engage to evaluate their work as a team. The team should agree on the purpose of the evaluation and intended users before approaching potential evaluators. Teams should meet with potential evaluators and share this information with them prior to selecting an external evaluator or evaluation team. Good evaluators will challenge the team to clarify their purpose and clearly identify their intended users prior to beginning any evaluation process, and will spend time with the team to fully understand their work together.

If the purpose of the evaluation is development of the team, team members will want to choose an evaluator who has experience in recognizing and evaluating team stages of development. An evaluator who understands the trajectory of team development over time will realize that not all teams are developmentally at the "performing" level, and that in the normal trajectory of team development, some "storming" is natural. Evaluators without this knowledge can be detrimental to a team that is using this evaluation in a developmental way—and could be discouraged by an evaluator who does not recognize normal development and may be critical of the team's performance. If the purpose of the evaluation is to evaluate team functioning to enhance individual performance appraisals, the team will want to select evaluators who understand and recognize the importance of individual contributions to team success. And, if the team's purpose in seeking external evaluation is an end-point evaluation to determine what could be learned from this team to enhance teamwork in the future in the organization, the team will want to select an evaluator who has a "big picture" perspective, and can evaluate the team in a way that will be readily translatable to other teams in the organization.

In selecting external evaluators, the team will also want to consider the intended users of the evaluation results. If the intended users are the team members only, evaluators should have a focus on the internal structure and functionality of the team. If the intended users are sponsors of the team or leaders in the organization, the evaluators will need to have a broader organizational context, providing these leaders with perspective on how the organization is facilitating or limiting the work of the team together.

Selecting external evaluators based on their knowledge of the team or their work together is an important consideration for team members. In some cases, selecting an evaluator within the organization (but outside of the team) may be an advantage to the team. An understanding of the organizational context of the work of the team may be helpful for the evaluator. Insights into the culture within which the team works, political pressures, organizational structures, and communication patterns may be invaluable in evaluating the progress of the team in their work together. However, evaluators within the same organization as the team may have some of the same issues with objectivity as team members do in performing self-evaluation. Personal relationships with team members, organizational loyalty, and preconceived notions of the need for the team's work together may influence evaluation processes by evaluators internal to the organization.

If objectivity is an issue, team members may want to choose an evaluator external to the organization. There are a number of commercial entities that perform this work for teams. Typically, the evaluators are trained in a model of evaluation that may be proprietary to the organization for which they work, or they may use standardized measures of team success in their evaluation. The advantage that teams have with using an external evaluator lies in the experience of these evaluators, their training in team evaluation, their experience with a variety of teams and organizations, and their ability to look objectively at team functioning without any of the influences that can challenge an evaluator internal to the organization. That said, the use of an external evaluator may be expensive, both financially and in human costs. Typically, external evaluators will need to spend more time with the team to understand not only the purpose of the evaluation but also the organizational context within which they function. Although there are ways to decrease financial costs, the importance of the investment of time in working with external evaluators to completely understand the work of the team together cannot be underestimated. Consider the following case example of how a team selected and used an external evaluation team to enhance their work together:

> A team of statewide partners from a variety of health care organizations came together in 2004 to develop a leadership institute for the development of emerging nurse leaders statewide. The purpose of the partnership was to not only govern the leadership institute but also to develop a partnership that could work together as a team outside of this program for problem solving in other areas of their common work. To evaluate their work together as a team in both the governance of the program and in their work together as a continuing partnership outside of the leadership institute, the team first considered the choice of evaluators. Because this partnership spanned organizational boundaries, the team agreed that evaluation by any entity within any one of their organizations could potentially introduce bias into the evaluation process. The partners therefore agreed to engage an external evaluation group to provide them with an evaluation of their work together and insights into opportunities for their future development as a team. Because funds were limited, the partners began to look at ways to facilitate a high-quality external evaluation while controlling costs. The partnership learned of a local university graduate business program that assigned teams of students working on their masters of business administration degree to gain real-life experiences in working with organizations to solve their business dilemmas. After meeting with the university faculty, the partnership was selected as a "company" to be assigned a student evaluation team. The external evaluation team first met with the team leaders to clarify the purpose of the evaluation, the scope of the evaluation (which was focused only on the team partnership, not on evaluation of the program they were governing), and the intended users of the evaluation. The student evaluators examined a variety of partnership documents provided by the team, including reports of their work together, meeting minutes, and other documents. The student evaluators attended partnership meetings and observed the work of the partners together. Focus groups of small groups of partners were convened,

and partnership-specific surveys were developed to collect impressions of the teams' actual and potential work together outside of the governance of the institute. Individual interviews with team members were undertaken to ascertain specific examples of how the partnership worked together, the barriers to their collaboration, as well as opportunities for future collaboration. Visits to individual organizations by the evaluators allowed them to see firsthand how the partnership was benefiting the mission of individual organizations involved in the partnership, and the environments within which the partnership was functioning. Case studies of successes, barriers, and future opportunities were developed to demonstrate how the partnership had worked together successfully, and where opportunities existed to improve the partnership and take advantage of emerging situations where the existing partnership could impact patient care and workforce development. The evaluation team presented its results to the partners with clear recommendations for future growth and a recommendation comparison to allow the partners to see the potential of each recommendation to sustain and grow the partnership.

This exemplar clearly identifies the value of external evaluation under the right circumstances, with a motivated team and the right evaluators. Creativity in selecting an evaluation team allowed the partnership to gain the expertise of the graduate students, who all came from outside of the health care environment and brought different perspectives to this evaluation. The students were supervised by faculty who were experts in their field, and that expertise was translated into the evaluation process. The partnership was clearly invested in the evaluation and took the time to participate in the variety of evaluation techniques that were used to tease out how the partners could work together more effectively in the future. All of these elements led to a successful evaluation and a strengthened partnership.

STANDARDIZED MEASURES FOR TEAM EVALUATION

In Chapters 2 and 3, we discussed a number of evaluation tools for individual team members. These tools were focused on identifying individual team member preferences for teamwork, their skills, talents and knowledge, and their competencies. These tools can be used to develop the team for success. Once a team has been developed, standardized evaluation measures can also be helpful in evaluating the team's functioning, identifying gaps in performance and suggesting strategies for improvement for the future.

Many standardized team evaluation measures exist. A few team evaluation survey measures will be reviewed here. A web search will reveal many different surveys. Selection of these measures is a complex undertaking and requires attention by the team for the purpose of the evaluation, what the team wishes to examine in the evaluation, and how it will use the evaluation in the team's own development. Cost may be a factor in the selection of standardized team evaluation measures as well. Each measurement tool provides different insights for the team, and each will have features that the team may need for future development, such as recommendations for strategies to enhance performance. The team should carefully evaluate available tools prior to implementation as an evaluation measure.

CAMPBELL–HALLAM TEAM DEVELOPMENT SURVEY

The Campbell–Hallam™ Team Development Survey (TDS) (Campbell & Hallam, 1994) provides team feedback to improve team effectiveness and help them to reach their maximum potential. The survey addresses how team members feel about issues such as interpersonal interaction within the group, innovations, organizational support, and mission clarity. Survey results provide objective information on the team's strengths and weaknesses and can create a framework for effective change to help team members improve morale, productivity, and communication. The TDS results can help teams identify their strengths and weaknesses, assess and improve team effectiveness, benchmark team progress, strengthen team-building efforts, support total quality management, and continuous improvement initiatives. Based on years of careful research, the TDS survey authors have identified 19 aspects of team functioning critical to team effectiveness. These dimensions are grouped around four major themes, including resources (time and staffing, information, material resources, organizational support skills, commitment, skills), efficiency (mission clarity, team coordination, team unity, individual goals, empowerment), improvement (team assessment, innovation, feedback, rewards, leadership), and team success (satisfaction, performance, overall index).

The report received by TDS users has high utility in understanding team strengths and areas for improvement. A report that is generated for the team outlines the areas in which team members most agree on their performance, and where their assessments of their performance diverge. Team strengths are outlined, areas worth celebrating are highlighted, and areas for improvement, along with clear actions the team might take to improve are included. For instance, a team may find that it believes that it is working well together, but there is room for improvement in particular areas. Team strengths might be identified, such as the team has challenging goals for its work together, it has a clear purpose, the leader is skilled at leading the team, and the team understands how it works out disagreements. Problem areas might be identified by the team in specific areas, such as the need for a particular piece of equipment or resource to facilitate its work, or a need for a communication plan outside of the team. The team may have identified that its focus is too scattered, and so it needs to focus on fewer tasks. Based on these problems, the TDS tool provides the team with some suggestions for improvement. These may include actions like presenting the case for the new piece of equipment or resource to the team sponsor or organizational administration, developing strategies for communication outside of the team, or working together to select the highest priority tasks needing the team's attention, and develop a plan for team emphasis on those items.

The team can choose to use this feedback in any way it sees fit. Most teams will craft a continuing team development plan based on TDS results, and use that plan to guide its actions in the months after the assessment. The value of feedback like that provided in the TDS is that it is team centered, that all members of the team have an opportunity to provide input, and that the results provide specific direction for team action.

COMPREHENSIVE ASSESSMENT OF TEAM MEMBER EFFECTIVENESS

The Comprehensive Assessment of Team Member Effectiveness (CATME) was developed for the purpose of collecting peer and self-evaluations by team members based on extensive university research. Developed with a grant from the National Science Foundation, this tool is currently free for instructional use in educational settings. The functionality and language of the system are customized for educational settings, and no commercial version of the system exists at this time (www.catme.org). This may be an effective tool for nurse educators to use in the evaluation of student or faculty teams.

A web-based survey at www.catme.org makes it possible to collect data on team-member effectiveness in five areas. Users can configure the site to survey any or all of the areas of interest in the evaluation of teamwork effectiveness. These areas include:

1. Contributing to the team's work
2. Interacting with teammates
3. Keeping the team on track
4. Expecting quality
5. Having relevant knowledge skills and abilities

The CATME instrument is a behaviorally anchored rating scale that describes behaviors that are typical of various levels of performance in each of the five categories. Raters select the category of behaviors that most closely matches the actual behavior of each person on their team (including themselves). A sample instrument on the CATME website shows the behavioral descriptions for all five categories and allows users to test the system. Results are available by cohort or by individual. Figure 7.1 demonstrates a cohort or team report, and Figure 7.2 an individual report.

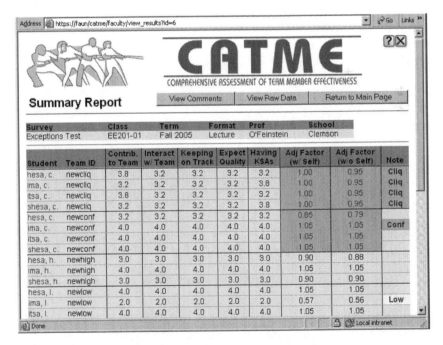

FIGURE 7.1 CATME aggregate results.

Source: Reprinted with permission of Ohland (2012). Retrieved from http://www.catme.org

Interacting With Teammates

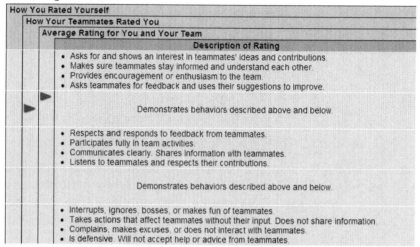

How You Rated Yourself			
	How Your Teammates Rated You		
		Average Rating for You and Your Team	
			Description of Rating
			• Asks for and shows an interest in teammates' ideas and contributions. • Makes sure teammates stay informed and understand each other. • Provides encouragement or enthusiasm to the team. • Asks teammates for feedback and uses their suggestions to improve.
			Demonstrates behaviors described above and below.
			• Respects and responds to feedback from teammates. • Participates fully in team activities. • Communicates clearly. Shares information with teammates. • Listens to teammates and respects their contributions.
			Demonstrates behaviors described above and below.
			• Interrupts, ignores, bosses, or makes fun of teammates. • Takes actions that affect teammates without their input. Does not share information. • Complains, makes excuses, or does not interact with teammates. • Is defensive. Will not accept help or advice from teammates.

FIGURE 7.2 CATME individual results by self, peers, and team.

Source: Reprinted with permission of Ohland (2012). Retrieved from http://www.catme.org

FREE STANDARDIZED SURVEYS

A quick web search for team evaluation surveys will likely produce a number of free surveys for team evaluation. The same criteria for selection of these surveys as is used for selecting other surveys can be applied by teams in selecting one of these tools for evaluation. Teams should remember that the questions in these surveys may not be backed by research, nor may they be applicable to the team's purpose. However, using a standard, web-based team survey might meet the team's needs, and could be a helpful adjunct to other forms of evaluation. A free template for a team evaluation survey that asks team members questions regarding understanding of team goals, resources, feedback, contributions of team members, and conflict resolution is available at www.123contactform.com/free-form-templates/Team-Evaluation-37436.

SUMMARY AND NEXT STEPS

The evaluation of the performance of a team is essential for the future development of the team as well as for the development of other teams in the organization. Teams must have a clear intention when they evaluate their work together. Carefully considering the purposes of evaluation, including individual performance appraisal, team development, or analysis of lessons learned for future teams, will help the team to select the appropriate timing of the evaluation and the type of evaluation most appropriate to the purpose. Teams can choose self-evaluation or evaluation by a person or group external to the group or organization, and can use a variety of methods to gather data for evaluation, including commercially available evaluation instruments. Regardless of the way teams evaluate their performance, the elements of commitment, trust, purpose, communication, involvement in the team, orientation to team processes, and dedication to continuous improvement should serve as the guiding framework for the team in its evaluation. In the next chapter, we will learn how to maintain team engagement through careful use of team evaluation, understanding what makes a team thrive, and how team leaders can infuse these elements into the work of their teams.

QUESTIONS FOR THOUGHT

1. Analyze your current team for Eickenberry's (2007) key elements of team success, including commitment, trust, purpose, communication, involvement, process orientation, and continuous improvement. Provide examples of how your team meets or does not meet expectations in each of these areas.
2. Plan a team self-evaluation. How might you involve all team members in the evaluation? How can you use the results of team self-evaluation to improve team effectiveness?
3. Consider how your team might use external evaluation to improve its effectiveness. What are some advantages for your team in using external evaluators? How might you creatively engage external evaluators of your team? How would you work with external evaluators to facilitate their work with your team?
4. Analyze some commercial measures for team evaluation for utility in evaluation of your team. What are the advantages of using one or more of these measures? What are the limitations to using one or more of these measures in your team's environment?

Nursing and Health Care Team Issues and Challenges

EIGHT

Periodic Maintenance for Thriving Nursing and Health Care Teams and Partnerships

Coming together is a beginning. Keeping together is progress. Working together is success.
—Henry Ford

LEARNING OBJECTIVES

1. Describe what elements stimulate a team to thrive.
2. Analyze team motivators and stimulators.
3. Identify ways to nurture a creative environment for teams.
4. Describe creative methods for brainstorming that can be used for team success.
5. Understand the conditions under which it might be necessary to disband a team.

Maintaining any relationship is hard work. Consider relationships in your personal or professional lives. Personalities, emotions, distance, and energy may all enter into your ability to maintain relationships. Consider these difficulties and how they may be compounded with a team or partnership, brought together under circumstances that may be tentative, temporary, or even crisis-like. Team leaders are challenged not only to keep teams working together toward a common goal but also to thrive in a creative environment while accomplishing their work together. Maintaining and facilitating engagement is essential for team success. But how can leaders accomplish continual engagement of their team? How can they engage team members in the leadership and followership paradigm within the team? And, when is it time to let go? This chapter will provide insights into what makes a team thrive, how to infuse strategies for motivation into your team while promoting and reaffirming the team's purpose, how to spark creativity, and finally, how to know when to let go—of the team, or of an individual member or members. Embracing these skills will help leaders keep their team energized for continued work together, even over the long term.

WHAT MAKES A TEAM THRIVE?

Think back to the best team you ever were a part of, in either your personal or professional life. What made that team thrive? How did that team stay together and work effectively throughout its lifespan? Many team members will say things like "we were constantly challenged," or "our work mattered." Others will say "we were able to direct ourselves in our work," or "we felt like we had a purpose," or "we knew what we wanted to achieve." Still others will mention leadership, and talk about the leader's skills, experience, or ability to motivate. Finally, team members will talk about how they had the skills they needed to accomplish their goals. They felt a sense of mastery and accomplishment. They were motivated to persist at their work. The literature supports these observations by team members. In his book *Drive: The Surprising Truth About What Motivates Us*, Pink (2009) found that today's workforce is motivated by three factors: autonomy, mastery, and self-direction. Pink provides leaders with a variety of motivating exercises that go beyond the traditional reward-and-punishment system or pay-for-performance system that is so often used in the workplace today. Based on decades of studies of motivation, Pink suggests that strategies to increase autonomy, mastery, and self-direction in the workplace and in life should support an intrinsic motivation that is not based on any external "carrot and stick" system of traditional motivation.

Research in health care has found similar results with regard to motivation. Edgar (1999) used the Job Characteristics Model of Work Motivation (Hackman & Oldham, 1976) to analyze job motivators for nurses in Canada. Hackman and Oldham (1976) suggest that the core job dimensions of *skill variety, task identity, task significance, autonomy,* and *feedback* are work motivators. According to Hackman and Oldham, *skill variety* involves the degree to which the work necessitates a variety of different activities that require diverse skills and talents. *Task identity* is the degree to which completion of work involves a whole and identifiable piece of work. *Task significance* is the degree to which the work impacts the lives of others. *Autonomy* in Hackman and Oldham's model involves the degree of independence, freedom, and self-direction involved in the work. Finally, *feedback* involves the degree to which the individual received clear and direct feedback about performance. Findings of Edgar's (1999) study supported the applicability of the Job Characteristics Model to the work of nursing. Edgar also found that *support for autonomy* by peers and leaders contributed significantly to motivation for nurses.

In a literature review of motivation and nursing, Toode and colleagues (2011) reviewed 24 nursing research studies on motivation and found that although neither clear understanding nor consensus about the concept of work motivation has been reached in the nursing literature, categories of factors affecting the work motivation of nurses can be identified and include:

- Workplace characteristics
- Working conditions
- Personal characteristics
- Individual priorities
- Internal psychological states

The encouraging finding for teams and team leaders from Toode and colleagues' (2011) review is that each of these factors is either intrinsic to the work environment (workplace characteristics, working conditions) and can be controlled by a team leader, or intrinsic to the person (personal characteristics, individual priorities, internal psychological states) and team members can be selected for these positive motivating factors. Both the positive workplace and individual characteristics can be changed, developed, facilitated, and nurtured by the team and team leader.

In a study of medical surgical nurses in Cyprus, Lambrou, Kontodimopoulos, and Niakas (2010) found that *achievements* were ranked first among four motivators by nurses, followed by *remuneration*, *coworkers*, and *job attributes*. Lambrou and colleagues, like other researchers, concluded that health care professionals tend to be motivated more by intrinsic factors, implying that intrinsic factors should be a target for effective employee motivation.

How can all of these studies be applied to the work of teams in health care? How can we use this evidence to allow our teams to thrive? Let us consider the main attributes of motivation posited by Hackman and Oldham (1976) and Edgar (1999) and apply them to teams. How can a team and a team leader remain motivated through the consideration of the concepts of *skill variety, task identity, task significance, autonomy, support for autonomy,* and *feedback*?

Skill Variety

Most of the work of teams requires skill variety. Typically, teams take on complex, system-based work that involves a variety of skills, talents, and competencies to be successfully completed. In Chapter 2, we discussed the selection of team members based on skills, skill gaps, and intentionally planning the work of the team to maximize skill use in the team. So, inherently, the work of teams involves skill variety. However, the role of the team leader should be to assure that all the skills available on the team are applied to the work of the team. Although team leaders have intentionally selected team members for their skills, it is the tendency of some teams to depend on a few people to apply their skills to do most to the work of the team. Taking time to think through how the variety of skills available to the team can be applied at different times in the work of the team is essential to keeping a team motivated. If a team member has a skill that is not being used at the current time, but will be needed in the future, keeping that team member motivated is especially important. Consider, for instance, the team member who has great strength in public speaking and winning others over with a persuasive style. Those skills may not come into play early in the team's work together, but rather will be essential when the team must present results, make recommendations based on its work, or secure additional resources. The leader must be sure that this team member understands when his or her skills will be most needed, but also tap into other skills of the team member during the early work of the team to keep him or her motivated.

Task Identity

Many times in health care, individual providers lack the opportunity to see the "whole" or an identifiable piece or work, in which they can see their contributions and have pride in accomplishment. Nurses in particular rarely see the "finished product" of patients they have cared for, since their time with a patient during the patient's contact with the health care system—a primary care visit, a hospitalization, or another episode of care—may be brief. It is difficult to remain motivated without being able to see the finished "whole," the fruits of the nurse's work with the patient in education, health promotion, or restorative functions are rarely seen by the nurse. The team, on the other hand, does have the opportunity to see its work through to its natural conclusion and to witness an identifiable piece of work. Even if the work of the team has multiple roadblocks, the team and team leader can work together to maintain their vision of the finished product. The team charter discussed in Chapter 4 can be a helpful way for teams to remain motivated to meet the mission identified in the team charter. Periodically revisiting that charter, reviewing the mission of the team, or keeping the mission and/or charter front and center at each team meeting may be a help. One team keeps its mission as a team front and center by placing the mission at the top of every team meeting agenda. Simple solutions to keeping the "eye on the prize" can be effective in motivation.

Task Significance

Linking the work of the team back to the overall mission of the organization is the most important way a team leader can facilitate motivation in the realm of team significance. The leader creates a culture within a team that relates to the significance of their work. The leader can consistently remind the team of the big-picture link between their work and the work of the organization. Storytelling related to the impact of the work of the team is a valuable and memorable way for a leader to maintain the focus on the significance of the work of the team. As suggested in Chapter 6, begin each meeting with a story of how the work of the team will impact a group of patients, the organization, or the community. Linkages back to the greater good are a powerful motivator for team members.

Autonomy

Autonomy appears as a key motivator in most studies of teamwork. The discretion to decide about the direction of the work, the strategies taken, and the actions that follow are essential to facilitating team satisfaction with the work. Although team leaders may have a more active role in the early stages of team formation (as discussed in Chapter 4), team leaders of more mature teams must learn to facilitate and guide the work of the team, as opposed to directing the work. As Edgar's (1999) research demonstrated, the support of autonomy is important in the motivation of nurses. Edgar suggested organizational changes that might support autonomy, including the "vertical loading of the job." This concept involves transferring responsibility and authority that was formerly held at higher levels in the organization to those who are actually doing the work. Shared governance is cited as a model of vertical loading, and can support autonomy in organizations (Edgar, 1999). In studying innovation teams, Hoegl and colleagues (2006) found that interference by leaders and team-external partners in the work of the team actually decreased the quality of work by the team. This should serve as a guide then for team leaders, who should endeavor to create a culture of autonomy in teams through providing team members with information rather than instructions and leading by assistance with goal setting and the provision of feedback rather than micromanaging the work of the team (Hoegl & Parboteeah, 2006).

Feedback

Feedback is simply about communication. We have stressed the importance of communication to team effectiveness throughout this chapter. The team leader can continually motivate teams to thrive through the

---

TABLE 8.1 The Traffic-Light Team Coaching Model

The process of the traffic-light team coaching model:

1. Give each team member a Post-it.
2. Write on the flip chart
   - Stop
   - Start
   - Continue
3. Explain that in a moment each member of the team will sit on the "hot seat" (put a seat out at the front of the room).
4. The rest of the team will then take turns to say one thing they would like this team member to "start, stop, and continue" doing.
5. Once on the "hot seat" that team member listens to the feedback (without comment).
6. Ask the team to look around the room and to start jotting down on each Post-it things they would like each member of the team to "stop, start, and continue" doing.
7. It is likely that this will cause discomfort to some of the team members. Explain that the feedback that they give is not "the truth"; it is just a perception. The person on the receiving end can choose to ignore or take on board the feedback.
8. Give the team 5 minutes to jot down some ideas.
9. Ask the first volunteer to take the "hot seat."
10. Ask the facilitator to take notes to record the comments.
11. Make sure the feedback is given and received without long stories, explanations, or apologies.

Source: Reprinted with permission of Liz Scott, Liz Scott Coaching. Retrieved from http://www.coachingconnect.co.uk

use of regular feedback. Informal and formal communication and feedback systems allow all members of the team to share how they think they are doing as a team. Leaders can help to organize feedback systems and provide encouragement, information about changing situations, and support to the team. Team leaders should remember that the purpose of feedback is to facilitate ongoing team development. Therefore, feedback needs to be supportive and enlightening. A technique suggested by Scott (2012) for providing supportive and enlightening feedback in a team is the "traffic light method." This method was adapted by Scott from the work of Myles Downey (2003). Each team member is requested to both give feedback and receive feedback. The feedback is facilitated by the team leader or a team sponsor. Scott suggests that this feedback process works best with small teams of six or fewer members. Because of the sensitive nature of feedback and the discomfort that some team members might feel during feedback sessions, careful selection of opportunities to use this technique must be considered. A debriefing session by the team leader or sponsor may be helpful if feedback is difficult for any member to receive. The steps in the model are found in Table 8.1.

SPARKING CREATIVITY IN TEAMS

Working in a creative environment can help teams to thrive, and nurturing a creative climate is important work of the team leader. Health care today calls for innovative thinkers to solve today's problems with tomorrow's solutions. Nurturing a creative and innovative environment requires getting past the common stumbling blocks of creativity. These barriers are described by Thompson (2003) as *social loafing, conformity, production blocking,* and *downward norm setting.* Thompson (2003) describes social loafing as the "tendency for people in a group to slack off, such as not work as hard either mentally or physically in a group as they would alone" (Thompson, 2003, p. 100). This can be a special problem for teams that have been together for a long time, or whose work together is slowed down or stopped by some external factor or factors. Keeping the team motivated and creative is especially difficult in these situations. *Conformity,* as described by Thompson, is the tendency for teams to respond to each other or to ideas in "appropriate" or traditional ways and in highly similar fashions throughout their work together. In short, team members want to be accepted by the others on their team, and so conform. A team leader is challenged to overcome this barrier while still providing some structure for the team, providing a safe place for divergent ideas to be discussed. *Production blocking* is a common threat to creativity in any work group. Especially in a team in which traditional brainstorming is occurring, group members may lose their creative thoughts while listening to others, or may be so focused on their thoughts that they do not take an opportunity to build upon the creative thoughts of others on the team. This is what Thompson terms *production blocking*: the tendency for idea production to be blocked during team brainstorming sessions (p. 101). Finally, *downward norm setting* is the thought that groups tend to regress toward the mean. In Thompson's terms, "the least productive members of the team are more influential in determining overall team performance than the high performers" (p. 101).

How does a team leader use knowledge of these barriers to develop and sustain over time a creative environment for their teams? There are a number of techniques that can lead to creative environments for teams, some of which can be used throughout the lifespan of a team, others of which need to be considered from the time of team selection.

Team Diversity

First, during team selection, and as we discussed in Chapter 2, the team leader should endeavor to assure that the team is diverse. Diverse backgrounds, educational credentials, professional experiences, skills, knowledge, personalities, and attitudes will lead to diverse thinking in the team, and will overcome some of the blocks to creativity, especially in the area of conformity. Team leaders should consider how the mix of team members will facilitate the creative environment for the team. In their report on diversity and innovation in the workforce, Forbes (2011) reports that the majority of over 300 chief executive officers (CEOs) surveyed recognized that diversity is a key driver of innovation and is a critical component of success. A diverse set of experiences, perspectives, and backgrounds is crucial to innovation and the development of new ideas. For firms that specialize in innovation and creative solutions to problems, like IDEO (www.ideo.com), a design firm that helps organizations innovate, teams are made up of members with broad expertise, from mechanical engineering to fine arts, and from a variety of generations, cultures, and backgrounds. In health care, the Center for Medicare and Medicaid Services (CMS) Innovation Center has empanelled a team of Innovation Advisors—recognizing the need for a diverse set of skills to aid with the testing and dissemination of innovations across the health care system. The Innovation Advisors Program brings together dedicated, diversely skilled individuals in the health care system to:

- Support the Innovation Center in testing new models of care delivery.
- Utilize their knowledge and skills in their home organization or area in pursuit of the three-part aim of improving health, improving care, and lowering costs through continuous improvement.
- Work with other local organizations or groups in driving delivery system reform.
- Develop new ideas or innovations for possible testing of diffusion by the Innovation Center.
- Build durable skills in system improvement throughout their area or region.

To learn more about the CMS Innovation Center Innovation Advisors program and how the lessons learned through this federal initiative can be transferred to local teams and organizations, team leaders can visit their website at www.innovations.cms.gov/initiatives/Innovation-Advisors-Program/index.html.

Fostering a Creative Environment

Fostering a creative environment takes planning. Amabile (1998) has been studying the facilitators of creativity for decades. Amabile developed the Intrinsic Motivation Principle of Creativity, positing that "people will be most creative when they feel motivated primarily by the interest, satisfaction, and challenge of the work itself, and not by external pressures" (Amabile, 1998, p. 79). Amabile identified six areas in which leaders hinder creativity. Not surprisingly, these factors align closely with those reviewed earlier that hinder motivation, and include challenge, freedom, resources, work-group features, supervisory encouragement, and organizational support. Although these are rarely the purview of only the team leader, and link back to the support, culture, and environment within the organization, the team leader can impact each of these areas in order to create a motivating environment and subsequently increase creativity in their teams.

Challenge: Team leaders can diminish the barriers in the area of challenge by matching team members to roles that challenge them. Matching team roles with team member skills is one way to accomplish this. However, some team members may also appreciate the opportunity to stretch beyond their current skill set and learn new skills. Team leaders can recognize the need for challenge within their teams and create opportunities for challenge to exist—effectively reenergizing the team for creativity.

Freedom: Team leaders can overcome barriers to creativity in the area of freedom by allowing the team to work independently while guided by a clear and consistent set of objectives. Team leaders who are cognizant of the team's stage of development will use this information to decide when to change their leadership role from one of a manager to one of a facilitator or guide. Increasing the freedom of the team to have authority over the work and work processes can lead to increased creativity.

Resources: If a team spends most of its time trying to find resources that it needs to do its work, the team's creativity potential plummets. These resources include physical resources like space, materials, access to the literature in the team's area of interest, and benchmarking data. Also included are human capital resources, like having staff support for the work of team that eats up their productive time, like scheduling of meetings, keeping minutes, and posting documents to shared sites. Probably the most important resource that any team leader can negotiate for his or her team is the intangible but essential resource of time. Team leaders can help to negotiate time for their team to work and be creative, and can also help the team to use its time productively through serving as a guide to the team.

Work-group features: As emphasized earlier, diversity in a team is key to its success. Team members need to be exposed to others who have different skills, ways of processing information, and thinking in order to be stimulated toward creativity. If the team has been created with heterogeneity in mind, different perspectives will lead to creative thinking.

Supervisory encouragement: A prime barrier to creativity is leaders who respond to new ideas skeptically, failing to acknowledge potential in new ideas. If a team spends more time trying to figure out which ideas the leader would not "shoot down" than it does trying to nurture its collective creativity, innovation and inventiveness will suffer. The team leader can develop a culture in which ideas are freely expressed, there is an open exchange of ideas, and evaluation of new ideas is a constructive process.

Designing the Work Environment for Creativity

Removing the barriers to creativity is a first step in the facilitation of team creativity. But how does a team leader foster creativity on a day-to-day basis? Most of us in health care do not have the luxury of designing our workspace for creativity from the ground up. Typically, we must make do with the space available to us for our team to use in its work. However, that does not mean that every meeting of the team must take place seated around a conference table. Team leaders can design the environment for creativity through using a few techniques gleaned from the most creative industries.

In a 2012 *Wall Street Journal* article, the emergence of stand-up meetings was examined (Silverman, 2012). Emerging as ways to start the day at many high-tech firms, stand-up meetings in this case are similar to the daily scrums discussed in Chapter 4. Stand-up meetings are just what they sound like, everyone stands up for the entire meeting—even if a member of the team is joining the team for a meeting virtually, he or she is required to stand up! What do stand-up meetings accomplish? Stand-up meetings diminish distraction. Without having a conference table, team members are less likely to have a laptop computer or a smartphone in front of them, distracting them from the work of the team and hence diminishing the collective creativity of the group. In terms of creativity, stand-up meetings can energize the group, facilitate more moving around and interaction, and create an alternative environment for creative thinking. Team leaders can adapt the stand-up meeting strategy for their teams. Plan to move all of the tables and chairs out of a meeting room on a day when the team plans to spend their time generating ideas. Use whiteboards, flip charts, or cover walls with paper and encourage participants to draw their ideas on the walls for everyone to gather around. Contrast the energy in this type of a meeting to that of a team meeting where everyone is sitting around a conference table—it is easy to see how creativity might increase in this energized environment.

Team leaders can also learn a lesson from creative environments like those developed at Google, Pixar, and Red Bull. A quick Internet search will provide team leaders with images of these workspaces—including the absence of cubicles, bright colors, shared workspace, and the focus on collaboration and fun—like sliding boards instead of stairs! The commonality among all of these workspaces is the unexpected. So, while as a team leader in a health care setting, you may not be able to install sliding boards in your workspace, you can create the unexpected. Gather your team for a meeting in a quiet waiting room where modular furniture can be pulled together to create a meeting space unlike a conference room. On a beautiful day, pull your flip chart outside. Paper the walls of your meeting space with the doodles of your team from a previous meeting. Plan a retreat day away from campus. Take a 2-hour lunch and watch a movie together while you eat. Create a physical environment that will stimulate your team to create!

BRAINSTORMING AND OTHER CREATIVE TECHNIQUES

Most people have participated in a traditional brainstorming session at some point or another in their lives. Traditional brainstorming has fallen out of favor in recent years, with opponents citing the prejudging or criticism of ideas during these sessions as an inhibitor of creativity. Fortunately, there are many alternatives to traditional brainstorming that can be used by teams and their leaders to stimulate creative thinking and to generate innovative ideas that may serve as seeds for their continued work together. A few key ground rules should be involved in any creative technique. These include:

1. *Judging is banned:* No criticisms or judgments should be made about anything that anyone says in a creativity session. Terms like "that's not a good idea" should be banned from the team's language.
2. *Freewheeling thought is encouraged:* No idea is too absurd to bring up to the team in any brainstorming technique. The leader can create a culture in which the wilder the idea the better, because it will open up new paths of thought for the team to explore. An idea that starts as *"we should develop a housing complex where only persons who have diabetes can live"* can eventually lead to creative thinking about group education for persons with diabetes, or innovations that affect the features of the care environment.
3. *Quantity is good:* The goal is always to come up with as many ideas as possible.
4. *Piggybacking is allowed:* As a new idea is brought up in the conversation, the team should be encouraged to build on that idea. If the team is using visual techniques, the team can begin to connect ideas on paper or a whiteboard with arrows or adjoining circles.
5. *Questions are good:* Not only are ideas important to the creative process, but questions are as well. Questions can be used to clarify (tell me more about that?) or to be provocative (is the way we currently educate nurses the best way?).

Some techniques that go beyond traditional freeform brainstorming are reviewed here. Team leaders can use any of these techniques in isolation or in combination at different points during the lifecycle of their teams.

Sketch Storming

Sketch storming is the graphical equivalent of brainstorming, in which ideas are sketched. The sketches are simple and quick, and they outline the idea or concept. In a recent sketch-storming session on how to motivate a team, one participant drew pictures of a variety of chocolates! In another session on how to engage young nurses in the organization, a participant drew a picture of a diploma and a trophy, indicating opportunities for continuing educational development and recognition as ways to engage her generation. The point is that everyone in the session understands the idea, and can build upon it through connecting other ideas and sketches.

World Café

A World Café (www.theworldcafe.com) is designed to develop conversations that explore questions that matter. The steps in a World Café session include clarifying the purpose of the session, creating a hospitable space, exploring questions that matter, encouraging everyone's contribution, connecting diverse perspectives, listening for insights, and sharing discoveries. The way a World Café is implemented is to have team members seated in small clusters (typically three to five people), and set up progressive rounds of conversation of about 20 to 30 minutes, depending on the complexity of the questions and the size of groups. Questions that matter to the team are posed to the cluster of team members. One member of the group is assigned to be the table host, and he or she introduces the question to the group and keeps the conversation flowing. Everyone is encouraged to write or draw ideas on their tablecloths (typically paper) so that the ideas can be shared with the next group that visits the table. After the allotted time has been reached, the team members move to a different table, with a different question for conversation. The table host welcomes the new team members and quickly shares the main ideas and themes from previous conversations. Team members are encouraged to link and connect their ideas to those of the past groups but also to bring new ideas and perspectives. Moving around and having conversations with different groups cross-pollinates ideas and insights. At the end of the session, team members can meet together to synthesize what they have discovered, ideas that they heard that are worth further exploration, and possibilities for future team action. A detailed guide called *Café to Go* is available for free download and distribution by team leaders with acknowledgment and reference to the link at www.theworld cafe.com. At a recent team meeting, the World Café technique was used and with 20 participants generated over 100 ideas in 90 minutes on how to empower employees within a large, multisite health care organization.

TABLE 8.2 SCAMPER Questions for Thought

SCAMPER VERB	TEAM QUESTIONS FOR THOUGHT
Substitute	What materials or resources can we substitute to improve the process? What other process could we use to reach the same outcome? What rules could we substitute for the current rules for this process? What will happen if we change our feelings toward this process (*especially for sacred cows*)?
Combine	What would happen if we combined this process with another process? What if we combined purposes or objectives? If we combined this process with another, how could we use our people differently?
Adapt	What other process is like this process? How could we adapt this process to mimic other processes? What other processes could we use for inspiration?
Put to another use	Who else could use this process? How would this process work in another setting? Organization?
Modify, magnify, or minify	What can we add to this process to modify it? Subtract? How could we change the process to make it more valuable?
Eliminate	What would happen if we stopped this process? How could we streamline the process? What steps in the process can we eliminate?
Reverse or rearrange	What would happen if we sequenced the steps in the process differently? How could we reorganize this process?

Source: Modified from MindTools (2012).

SCAMPER

In the early 1950s, Osborn, a pioneer in the study of creative thinking, wrote a book called *How To Think Up* (1952). In this book, he developed a list of action verbs that would lead to the generation of ideas about how to change something—a product or process, for instance. Later, Robert Eberle (1996) organized these action verbs into the acronym "SCAMPER." The verbs are:

- Substitute
- Combine
- Adapt
- Modify, magnify, or minify
- Put to another use
- Eliminate
- Reverse or rearrange

Using this technique can help a team to identify a multitude of possibilities for how to solve a particular problem. Questions the team can ask for each of the verbs in the SCAMPER method are found in Table 8.2.

If you apply each of these verbs to a procedure or situation that you would like to change, your team will come up with some creative ideas that could solve problems confronting the team.

USING THE LEADERSHIP–FOLLOWERSHIP RELATIONSHIP TO HELP A TEAM THRIVE

Most of this text has focused on how the leader of a team might use knowledge of teams and teamwork to intentionally develop, support, and facilitate the work of a team. However, in organizations, the work of followers is equally important to the work of leaders. In their recent analysis of the leadership–followership dynamic, Cox, Plagens, and Sylla (2010) state that "leadership is the capacity to exercise influence over the actions of others such that the others behave in the manner the leader desires. Leading is the self-conscious actions of an individual vested with the capacity and/or responsibility to exercise leadership. Traditionally, followership represents the conscious and unconscious behaviors of persons and groups in support of the goals and desires of a leader which have been expressed in words or conduct" (p. 38). So, in traditional terms, teams have leaders and followers. Leaders choose to lead, and followers choose to follow. The two roles are interdependent. However, Cox and his colleagues propose that followers are integral to organizational success, because they do not blindly obey organizational authority, but rather, they make a choice to follow an organizational or team leader based on relationships, shared goals, and interactions.

How can an understanding of team leadership and followership help a team to thrive? The concept of fluidity in the context of team leadership and followership is essential to understand. In recalling the team development model of Tuckman presented in Chapter 4, the team leader understands that the role of the team leader can fluctuate throughout the team's developmental process, from one of directing the work of the team, to one of facilitating the team's work when the team has matured. Taking this concept one step further, however, it is important to remember that at some point in the work of the team, alternate leaders may be essential for the team to thrive, and the former team leader may assume the role of follower; hence the fluidity of the relationship. Consider the following example of a team in which the leader assumed the role of follower to allow for team success:

> A hospital team that has been working together on the development of an alternative method for staff nurse promotion over the previous clinical ladder system has hit a stumbling point. The team leader, who has been effective in the development of the team and the facilitation of their work together on an innovative product for staff nurse promotion and recognition, is viewed in the broader organization as someone who is responsible for the previous promotion and recognition system, which has been the major satisfier of staff nurses in the organization for the last 5 years on every nursing satisfaction survey. The staff of the organization views the team leader as someone who is wedded to the old system, as someone who disregarded the dissatisfaction of the staff for many years, and someone who defended the old system in every forum. This mistrust of the team leader throughout the staff nurse ranks has spilled over into other initiatives led by this team leader, causing those initiatives to be met with resistance. Although the team has developed great respect and trust in the leader, the team is concerned that the general mistrust of the leader by the staff will cause this new promotion and recognition system to be met with great resistance and mistrust as well. The concern over the potential failure of their work is affecting the motivation of the team.

Because the team had developed clear and honest communication and mutual respect, a frank conversation was held at a team meeting. The viewpoints of team members who were concerned about project failure because of mistrust of the leader were presented in a nonconfrontational matter, and discussed rationally by the team and the leader. A plan for success was developed. The plan involved the team leader stepping into a follower role for the remainder of the project, with the team agreeing upon a new leader who had the trust of the team and staff, and would guide the team in the implementation and evaluation phase of their project. Team members celebrated the success of the team to this point, as led by the former team leader, and took actions to demonstrate the continued value of the former leader to the team.

In this example, these mature team members and leader demonstrated the common traits of teams presented in Chapter 1, including collective accountability and responsibility for their work, collaboration, open and frank communication, and shared decision making. They also understood the fluidity of the leadership–followership dynamic within their team. Through remembering these keys to success, the team was able to re-negotiate leadership and followership roles, increasing their motivation, and facilitating their continued success.

HOW TO KNOW WHEN TO LET GO

Despite the best efforts of a team leader to motivate, stimulate, and support a team, there are times in the development of a team when "adjourning," as discussed in Chapter 4, is the natural next step in the team's life cycle. How do team leaders know when it is time to let go?

For some teams, the time to let go is natural, the project for which they were formed is complete. In this instance, the role of the team leader is to help the team with the adjourning process—celebrating their successes (and failures for that matter!), cataloguing their accomplishments and what they have learned that can help future teams, and developing closure for the team. A final meeting of the team can accomplish all of these. Team leaders may want to think about how to make that final meeting special, to set it aside from previous meetings of the team. Some meet over lunch or away from the workplace for a final meeting. Still others plan a social event together to create closure; they attend a sporting event, a play, or a concert as their final work together. Team leaders may also want to acknowledge the contribution of the team in other ways—through a written communication to the sponsor detailing the team's successes, lessons learned, and thanking the team for their work, through writing an article about the team's work for a company blog or newsletter, or through the development of a short video spot highlighting the work of the team. The point for leaders is to acknowledge that the work of the team was special, and that the work made an impact on the organization.

It is more difficult for a leader to know when to let go of a team (or team member) when the work of the team is not complete. Sometimes teams and team members are just dysfunctional. Usually, those dysfunctional members or teams take up the majority of the time of the leader, taking the focus away from the intended work of the team. Although much has been written about turning around a dysfunctional team, little attention is given to the real-life problem of the dysfunctional team that is not worth further investment of time, energy, and resources. Clearly, there are times when the leader can no longer invest in the dysfunctional team—for instance, if the team has undertaken activities that are not legal or ethical. Immediate adjournment and other possible disciplinary actions within the organization are warranted. This is a rare occurrence. More likely, the team leader will be faced with a team that just does not meet its goals. Because organizations are depending on the team to meet a goal, the team that cannot meet its goals places the entire organization in jeopardy. Consider the dysfunctional team in the case below:

> An interprofessional team in a health sciences education program is brought together to develop an interprofessional core curriculum around safety and quality. The curriculum is to be designed for all health sciences learners, including medical, nursing, pharmacy, social work, public health, and allied health students. The team is carefully selected to represent all professions and to include those with skills from the clinical perspective as well as accomplished educators who have curricular development and evaluation expertise. Two co-leaders, a doctorally prepared nurse educator and a master's-prepared clinician educator, are appointed. The team spends time at the beginning of their work together to clarify their mission, to establish clear goals for their work

together, and to develop a plan for how they will move forward. About 6 months into their work together, trends that disrupt the work of the team begin to emerge. These include:

a. An acute focus by several of the members on the needs of their discipline over the needs of all learners.
b. A habit by several members of arriving near the end of meetings and disrupting the work accomplished by the team during the meeting by introducing their own new issues.
c. A power struggle related to leadership as one team member believes that he should have been appointed leader and begins to undermine the work of the team.
d. A generalized feeling of distress by the team related to their lack of progress.
e. Verbalization by team members of the burden of team meetings.
f. A trend toward the leaders doing the work of the team and the team supporting that trend.

The team leaders continually strategize and introduce team leadership strategies into their work. They facilitate communication, encourage autonomy, and provide resources. However, the team, after 12 months of work together, has not moved past the developmental stage of storming, and the only products produced by the team have been produced by the team leaders.

Despite all of the work put into selecting the right members, creating an environment of support replete with resources, and despite the leaders' best efforts at coaching, sometimes teams just cannot succeed. This team has demonstrated some of the key characteristics of team dysfunction, including lack of focus and accountability, individual members' focus on their own needs over those of the team, and inequitable distribution of work (Swyers, 2012). The decision of the team leaders, and eventually supported by the sponsors, was to disband the team. Sometimes this is the best response to a dysfunctional team— and in this case, the team members and leaders were relieved. Team leaders should consider disbanding a team with as much care and thought as they put into selecting and composing a team—although it seems counterintuitive, sometimes disbanding the team is the only way to make progress.

SUMMARY AND NEXT STEPS

The energy spent putting a team together, developing that team, maintaining its energy, and facilitating its creativity is energy well spent. Team leaders are challenged to keep a team moving toward a common goal while simultaneously thriving in a creative environment while accomplishing their work together. Leaders can use the knowledge and skills gained in this chapter to maintain and facilitat engagement for team success. In the next chapter, we will discuss how to continue to promote the team through leveraging the team's success both inside and outside of the organization. Getting the work of the team the attention it deserves and demonstrating the value of the team will be key skills necessary to allow the team to continue to thrive and succeed.

QUESTIONS FOR THOUGHT

1. What motivates your team? How do you use these motivators as a leader to help your team thrive in your organization? How are the concepts of skill variety, task identity, task significance, autonomy, support for autonomy, and feedback operationalized in your team? How can they be improved?
2. How would a feedback method, such as Scott's (2012) traffic-light method be received in your team? How as a leader might you introduce this method, or another method of feedback, to your team?
3. Are there barriers to creativity in your team? How do they appear in the work of your team? How do you as a leader remove these barriers?
4. How innovative is your team? What are some methods of sparking creativity that might be useful with your team, considering your team norms and organizational culture?
5. How fluid is the relationship between leaders and followers on your team? Are there times when the team leader must step aside to facilitate team motivation and success? Can you cite examples of this fluid dynamic between leaders and followers in current or past teams you have been involved with in your organization?
6. Consider the elements presented in this chapter that may be indicators of a need to disband a team. Have you ever been on a team or led a team that was disbanded? For what reason? How were the team's successes celebrated? If you as a team leader were faced with disbanding a team, what would be your strategy for adjournment?

NINE

Team Leadership Training and Development Program Exemplars

Spectacular achievements are always preceded by unspectacular preparation.
—Roger Staubach

LEARNING OBJECTIVES

1. Analyze components of successful team leadership training programs.
2. Identify situations in which team leadership training and development may be essential to a team's success.
3. Select components of successful team leadership training and development programs that will assist teams in developing team leadership competencies.
4. Evaluate team leadership training and development programs for suitability to the needs of the team.

A variety of team leadership development programs have been developed across the United States and the world. Teams and team leaders may find these formal programs helpful. Teams may find these programs helpful as teams are forming. However, established teams may find these programs to be integral to their future development as a highly functional team. Programs range from onsite interventions, web-based modules, to year-long onsite programs with teams practicing skills in their home organization over the course of the year. Some programs have specific foci, like patient safety or medication administration; others are general team development curricula, in which the training can be applied to a variety of team missions. In this section, a variety of team training program exemplars will be provided. One has been developed by the author, and is presented in full as a model team training program. Others are proprietary programs, and summaries of those programs are provided, along with links to the programs for readers to find out more about how to access these programs for use in their organizations. Teams should evaluate their needs for training, and match those needs to available programs. Teams may also select to choose parts of each of these programs based on training needs, and develop their own program.

Regardless of the format for a team training program, common content should be included in any curricula. The curricula should be designed to develop knowledge, skills, and attitudes related to teamwork for all participants. The Agency for Health Care Research and Quality (AHRQ) has suggested a framework for team training programs that could be a helpful model for those planning to develop a team training program, or for evaluating team training programs. The framework includes tools, methods, and strategies that could be used during a team training program to develop teamwork competencies. Key to the success of team training in this model is the ability of team members to self-analyze and correct, to practice skills, and to receive feedback in the safety of the training environment. Figure 9.1 shows the teamwork training framework suggested by AHRQ.

TEAM LEADERSHIP DEVELOPMENT PROGRAM EXEMPLARS

Team leadership development programs typically provide a variety of didactic lectures, self-learning modules, and other resources to increase knowledge. Practice of those skills then occurs in the team's home organization. The idea behind these programs is the immersion of participants in learning about teams and teamwork concepts, while enabling them to implement that learning with the support of programs and program faculty as they are working in their home organization. Teams develop knowledge, skills, and attitudes relative to teamwork, and practice to develop competencies in their organizational environment, adapting their work to that environment. Four program exemplars are summarized here, along with contact information to allow readers to access those programs and their resources to meet their own team training needs.

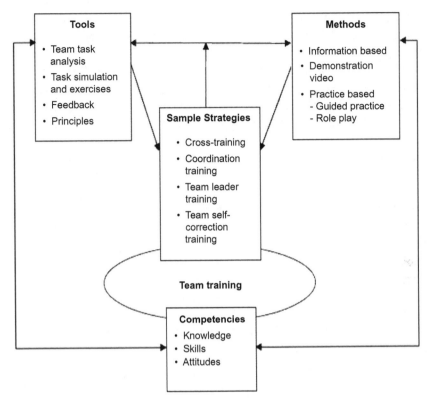

FIGURE 9.1 Framework for designing an effective team training program.
Source: From Cannon-Bowers and Salas (2000). Reprinted with permission of the American Psychological Association.

THE WEST VIRGINIA NURSING LEADERSHIP INSTITUTE

The West Virginia Nursing Leadership Institute (WVNLI) is an exemplar of a 1-year team development program. The mission of the WVNLI team development program is to prepare teams of nurses to effectively lead transformation in their organizations, communities, and beyond. WVNLI was developed with the understanding that teamwork has positive effects in health care organizations, especially in quality and safety of care. This includes reducing medical errors, improving quality of patient care, addressing workload issues, building cohesion, and reducing burnout of health care professionals. Improved communication, partnerships, clarity on the role of all health care providers, improved coordination of health care services, and high satisfaction for health care providers and patients are outcomes of effective teamwork.

Nurses who possess teamwork and leadership skills are sought for advancements in their career, enhancing their satisfaction, and influencing retention in the workplace. As the number of health care errors has risen in the United States, so has interest in the development of care delivery processes that minimize the potential for error. Among the strategies proposed by experts are the creation, training, and support of highly developed teams. With a nursing shortage threatening the quality of patient care, and currently being felt in all sectors of West Virginia health care, investment in team leadership and effectiveness skills is essential. For this reason, the West Virginia University School of Nursing—Charleston Division and the Charleston Area Medical Center Health Education and Research Institute collaborated to develop the WVNLI team development program to provide training in team leadership and effectiveness to teams of nurses from across West Virginia. Teams engaged in this 12-month program develop team leadership skills to shape the future of health care in their organizations and beyond.

The 12-month program allows team members to remain in their current positions while gaining the experiences, insights, networking, competencies, and skill enhancements necessary to effectively lead teams in the workplace and community.

The Program

The highly interactive Institute includes opportunities for teams to build and utilize team development and leadership skills, including:

- Building and maintaining effective teams
- Motivating and developing others and giving feedback
- Organizational analysis
- Strategizing, communicating with others, and planning
- Managing change
- Negotiation and conflict resolution
- Decision making
- Team focus and problem solving
- Measuring effectiveness through metrics

Teams of three to six nurses from each organization attend four intensive 2-day seminars over the course of 1 year. Intersession work includes web-based assignments and team leadership projects designed to offer solutions to challenges within the home organization. Teams receive ongoing support and mentorship from sponsors from the home organization and Institute faculty.

Eligibility Criteria

The program is open to teams of three to six registered nurses who work in any rural or urban health care agency, including hospitals, long-term care organizations, public health departments, primary care clinics, and schools of nursing. Ideal candidates are those teams that warrant investment by the employing agency because of their potential to impact change in their home organization. Home organizations identify issues in their environment that are amenable to intervention by a team, and purposefully select teams based on the needs they have identified. Teams are nominated and supported by the home organization during their team training and practice of team-based skills in the home organization.

Program Curriculum

The curriculum includes four 2-day sessions, three intersessions over the course of 1 year, and an alumni learning network. The program and topics covered during the program are as follows:

Onsite Session One—Team Models and Skills: During this introductory 2-day session, participants are introduced to the program, including expected outcomes. Participants are encouraged to explore their own team skills and needs, and through lecture, discussion, self-assessment, and evaluation, develop a plan for their team development. Expert consultant faculty guide teams in planning for their own development. Prior to this seminar, accepted participants will have completed assessment instruments, including the Myers–Briggs-Type Indicator (MBTI®; Myers, McCaulley, Quenk, & Hammer, 1998), and others. Using the MBTI results, teams develop a team profile, based on their preferences in the four dichotomies presented in Chapter 2, including extraversion/introversion, sensing/intuition, thinking/feeling, and judging/perceiving. Understanding characteristics unique to each personality type provides insight into how they influence an individual's way of communicating and interacting with others on the team. The tool is used by participants to identify their preferences relative to teamwork, and to formulate a team development plan. All of the self-assessment tools used in this seminar and throughout the Institute are designed to match team development strategies to individual and team preferences and behavior. Topics for lecture, discussion, and activities during this seminar include introduction to effective team models, preferences related to teamwork, team development, giving feedback within a team, dealing with conflict, organizational analysis as related to effective team work, and managing change as a team.

Intersession One—Problem Identification in the Home Organization: Intersession work continues building on team knowledge gained in onsite Session One. Each team has assignments to complete, develops an improvement plan for team development to guide them throughout the program, participates as a team with their organizational sponsor to identify a problem amenable to team intervention in the home organization, and participates in one live webcast provided by the program on a team development topic of interest or challenge to the participants. Alumni of the program also participate in the intersession webcast, allowing current participants to learn from an even larger community of teams.

Onsite Session Two: Taking Action/Program Planning: Session Two moves from development of the team to teamwork in the organization through the planning of a project amenable to team intervention, designed to impact on patient care quality, nurse satisfaction, and/or nurse retention. In this session, participant teams gain the tools needed to impact change within organizations. The impact of culture on individuals, teams, and organizations is stressed. Participants begin to plan for the implementation and evaluation of local projects in their home institutions. Use of a logic model for program planning is introduced. Appropriate metrics to evaluate effectiveness of the project are emphasized.

Intersession Two—Local Teamwork in Action: Planning, Implementation, Metrics, and Evaluation of Team Functioning: During intersession two, participants begin to practice team skills through implementation of a creative, organization-specific, patient care quality, nurse empowerment, nurse satisfaction, and/or nurse retention program in their home institution. In addition, teams are assisted in evaluating their team functioning and effectiveness at this midpoint in the team training through completion of the Campbell–Hallam Team Development Survey (TDS), as presented in Chapter 7. The TDS provides team feedback to improve team effectiveness and to help the team reach maximum potential. The survey addresses how team members feel about such issues as interpersonal interaction within the group, innovations, organizational support, and mission clarity. Survey results provide objective information on the team's strengths and weaknesses and can create a framework for effective change to help team members improve morale, productivity, and communication.

Onsite Session Three: Team Issues and Challenges: Teams continue development by building on strengths identified in the TDS, and applying knowledge to challenges such as fostering creativity, managing change, and thriving in a chaotic environment. During this session, team development specialists provide group review of feedback from the TDS, along with action planning for success. In addition, each team has an opportunity to participate in a 1- to 2-hour individual consultation relative to team strengths and development needs with team development specialists. Team members spend time reviewing their results and developing strategies for continued team development and success.

Intersession Three—Local Teamwork in Action: Evaluation: Participants begin to implement a plan to analyze the impact of their local projects using accepted evaluation metrics, begin to analyze the results of the project, and develop a plan for dissemination in their own institutions and with other participants. They attend a live webcast on a topic driven by their needs and provided by Institute faculty, and begin to mentor a team in their home institution, spreading their teaming skills throughout the organization.

Onsite Session Four—Team Results and Leverage: Participants share their team leadership and effectiveness successes and challenges. Participants also evaluate how they can continue to build an environment to facilitate team engagement in their workplace. Participants examine methods to leverage results of the development as a team and their projects both within the home organization and beyond. Topics such as selling upward and outward and coalition building, as well as next steps in their personal and team development, are discussed. Sponsoring institutional representatives and team sponsors are invited to participate in this session. In addition, key stakeholders in the state who can help with leveraging teamwork and results and coalition building for the future are invited to attend. These include representatives from the state nursing workforce center, local foundations, professional organizations, and government officials.

This intensive leadership development program has been tested with over 200 participants and success has been documented through self-evaluation of teamwork effectiveness, through evaluation by the sponsoring organization of the value of the team to the organization, and through external evaluations. Samples of evaluation data from one cohort of teams are presented in Table 9.1.

In addition, team participants were asked to rate their skills in certain team activities key to successful work. These ratings are consistently high, and demonstrate the impact of the program curriculum on nursing teams (Table 9.2).

End-of-program reports provide many additional insights into what the teams were able to accomplish and the impact of their work as a team on their local organizations. Whether the impact is measured in financial terms or in impact on human capital, all translate to improved patient experiences and outcomes. One team that worked to increase HCAHPS (Hospital Consumer Assessment of Healthcare Providers and Systems) and Press-Ganey scores regarding communication around medications in their organization reported *"we realized potential cost savings by increased patient satisfaction by increasing HCAHPS scores ... in turn increasing revenue for the hospital."* The program has also

TABLE 9.1
Self-Reported Impact of WVNLI Program on Team Leadership and Effectiveness Skills

SKILL	AVERAGE (1–5 SCALE, 5 = HIGHEST IMPACT)	STANDARD DEVIATION
Communication with others	4.31	0.97
Project management	4.25	1.11
Building and maintaining effective teams	4.19	0.94
Problem solving	4.16	0.95
Strategizing	4.16	0.94
Organizational analysis	4.13	0.87
Giving feedback	4.09	0.82
Motivating and developing others	4.03	0.78
Decision making	4.03	1.09
Measuring effectiveness through metrics	3.97	1.0
Negotiation and conflict resolution	3.78	1.29

$N = 32$.
Source: Persily (2010).

TABLE 9.2
Self-Assessed Team Activity Ratings

SKILL (1–5 WITH 5 = HIGHEST SKILL RATING)	RATING	STANDARD DEVIATION
Open communications/creativity	4.33	0.65
Listening	4.33	0.65
Team purpose	4.25	0.97
Positive feedback	4.67	0.65
Member communication	4.42	0.79
Conflict management	4.42	0.79
Decisions	4.42	0.79
Results	4.25	0.75
Organizational climate	3.75	0.97
Team rating	4.42	0.67
Member contribution	3.67	1.23
Team meetings	4.0	0.95
Change (impact)	4.25	0.75
Participation and leadership shared	3.5	0.90

$N = 32$.
Source: Persily (2010).

had an impact beyond the individual and team. Some of the key points that the program has helped developers learn and that could be helpful to others in planning similar programs include:

- Ideas for solutions to problems in health care organizations were seeded at other organizations as a result of the learning community established in the program. Teams learn from each other; strategies to facilitate learning from one another should be supported.
- Learning collaboratives are developed across teams, but also across cohorts and across sponsors as the alumni network grows statewide. Sponsors value the statewide network, which they can access to learn from other organizations how they have addressed similar challenges.
- Momentum for team leadership development in organizations is built through team projects. As projects are disseminated throughout an organization, more nurse leaders begin to desire participation in the program.
- Leadership and teaming translate beyond the walls of the institution to the community (Persily, 2010).

Organizations and teams that are interested in learning more about the WVNLI TDP can visit the home page at www.wvnli.org where additional program information, past team projects, and program evaluation data can be found.

TEAMSTEPPS

Another exemplar of team training is the TeamSTEPPS program, developed over the last 20 years by the Department of Defense's Patient Safety Program in collaboration with the AHRQ (www.teamstepps. ahrq.gov/about-2cl_3.htm). The program uses an evidence-based curriculum to impact team effectiveness, communication, and patient safety in health care organizations. The TeamSTEPPS model develops knowledge, skills, and attitudes that influence team outcome success in four areas. These areas include leadership, communication, mutual support, and situation monitoring. This team training addresses many of the topics that are presented in this chapter, with the targeted focus on patient safety as an outcome (Figure 9.2).

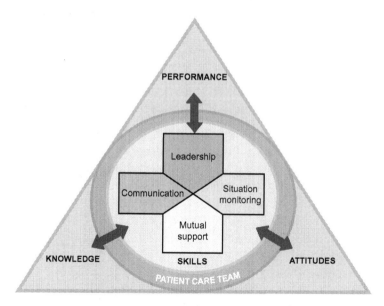

FIGURE 9.2 TeamSTEPPS[R] model.

Source: From TeamSTEPPS[®] model. Reprinted with permission of the Agency for Healthcare Research and Quality. Retrieved from www.teamstepps.ahrq.gov/teamsteppslogo.htm

TeamSTEPPS is implemented in a three-phase process that is designed to create and support a culture of safety that includes pre-training assessment for organizational readiness, a train-the-trainer program for onsite trainers and for health care providers, as well as support for implementation and sustaining the culture of safety.

Pre-Training Assessment

Health care organizations are provided with an opportunity to identify readiness of the organization for a change in safety culture in areas such as leadership support, identifying real or potential barriers to implementing a change in culture, and deciding whether crucial resources are in place for support of the initiative. This assessment includes a number of critical steps, which will be familiar to the readers:

- *Establish a change team:* This organizational-level team should be multidisciplinary and represent all categories of health care professionals within the organization. Successful change teams are comprised of organizational leaders who are committed to changing the current culture.
- *Conduct a site assessment:* This team training needs analysis and is a process used in TeamSTEPPS to systematically identify teamwork deficiencies, so training programs can be developed. This information is then used to identify critical training and develop training objectives.
- *Define the problem, challenge, or opportunity for improvement:* In this phase, the team is charged with identifying a problem that threatens patient safety and then determine how this problem results from existing processes and procedures. The team uses a variety of tools, including mapping, to identify the need for intervention in the organization.
- *Define the goal of the team intervention:* The team develops goals that will reduce or eliminate the risk to patient safety posed by the problem that it has identified. Specific tools for goal development and identification of responsibility and time limits are provided. During this phase, teams develop team process goals, team outcome goals (to reflect their development as a team), and a clinical outcome goal that reflects an increase in patient safety.

Implementation and Action Plan

The next step in the process identified by TeamSTEPPS is to develop an implementation and action plan, followed by training and implementation in the organization. The steps for planning, training, and implementation are:

- *Define the TeamSTEPPS intervention:* Teams decide, based on their organizational environment, whether "whole training" (all the tools in one sitting) or "dosing" (specific tools targeted to specific interventions) is the best intervention plan for their organization. Each of these methods has advantages and disadvantages, and the team is supported in decision making relative to training throughout the process.
- *Develop a plan for determining the intervention's effectiveness:* In Chapter 7 of this book, a variety of ways to assess teamwork and the impact of training were provided. In the TeamSTEPPS program, a variety of ways to evaluate the impact of training are provided. Teams develop a plan to evaluate whether team members have acquired new knowledge, skills, or attitudes at the end of training, how they are implementing that training, and organizational outcomes that have been impacted by team training.
- *Develop an implementation plan:* The team decides what groups in the organization need to be trained, and a plan for training that makes sense for the organization.
- *Gain leadership commitment to the plan:* Teams work with organizational leaders to gain the resources needed to implement the plan, and to refine the implementation plan as appropriate.
- *Develop a communication plan:* As discussed in Chapters 5 and 9, communication of the work of the team is essential. Critical to the success of any change is an understanding of the goal of the intervention by all involved; teams develop a plan to assure that all stakeholders understand their purpose.
- *Prepare the organization:* TeamSTEPPS advocates for team involvement in readying the organizational environment for the new tools and strategies gained during training to be transferred to their work environment.

Implement Training in the Organization

Teams begin to train the stakeholders in the environment with curricula designed to facilitate culture change through team training.

The TeamSTEPPS curriculum is a comprehensive multimedia kit that contains:

- Fundamental modules in text and presentation format
- A pocket guide that corresponds with the essential version of the course
- Video vignettes to illustrate key concepts
- Workshop materials, including a supporting CD and DVD, on change management, coaching, and implementation

Once the team has trained stakeholders to work as teams to improve care and patient safety, several steps are provided to sustain that change in the organization. These steps include providing opportunities to practice skills, ensuring that leaders emphasize new skills for teams, providing regular feedback and coaching, celebrating wins, measuring success, and periodically updating the plan based on changing organizational needs.

Organizations and teams that are interested in implementing a TeamSTEPPS intervention in their organizations can find out more about the program by visiting the TeamSTEPPS website at www.teamstepps .ahrq.gov. More tools, information about implementation, and program outcomes are available on this site.

GERIATRIC INTERDISCIPLINARY TEAM TRAINING

The Geriatric Interdisciplinary Team Training (GITT) program was developed by the John A. Hartford Foundation, Inc. and built on knowledge gained from the Veterans Administration Interdisciplinary Team Training Program in Geriatrics (Baldwin, 1996; Fulmer, Flaherty, & Hyer, 2003). The program was developed to meet a need for teams in the care of older adults in an era of increasing health care costs for this fragile population, cost containment, and managed care. Changes in the health care system in the mid-1990s required all team members to understand the knowledge, skills, and competencies of all providers on the team, and to coordinate care for older patients. Shifts to chronic disease models of care emphasize the importance of team care for older adults.

The GITT goals included the development of national training models for teams caring for older adults while strengthening partnerships between educators and clinicians, developing well-tested curricula for team training, increasing the number of providers of care for older adults who possess team competencies, and to test models of training for team care of older adults (Fulmer et al., 2003). The curriculum for this program includes topics such as teams and teamwork, roles and responsibilities, communication, conflict resolution, care planning processes, multiculturalism, and ethics for teams. The program has been implemented across the United States, with partnerships thriving between academic and clinical partners.

Readers who would like more information about the GITT program can visit their website at www.gittprogram.org. The website has case studies, sample teaching tools, assessment measures, and access to videos, team training materials, books, and more to facilitate team training to improve the care of older adults.

MEDTEAMS

MedTeams® is a team training program that has been developed by Dynamics Research Corporation, using lessons learned from the aviation industry's Crew Resource Management systems (Morey et al., 2003; Baker et al., 2005). The curriculum consists of 8 hours of classroom instruction in a train-the-trainer format. Learning modules and videos enhance the training. Once trainers have been trained, practica in teamwork, coaching for improving team behaviors, mentoring for teamwork competency, and review sessions are used to continue learning experiences for the team. One of the key elements for success of this program is the expectation of specific responsibilities at chief executive officer (CEO), director, and department levels for supporting the program. This element of the program is consistent with the discussion of the importance of team sponsors and mentors in Chapter 2. Measurement tools have been developed to evaluate the success of the team training intervention. This program has been used across the United States, originating in emergency departments, but now used in labor and delivery suites, operating rooms, and intensive care units.

Readers who are interested in learning more about the MedTeams program for their organization should visit the website www.teams. drc.com/Medteams/home/home.htm. Links to program examples, evaluation, and descriptions can be found at this site.

SUMMARY AND NEXT STEPS

Team training is necessary for teams to thrive in an organization. Building curricula to develop knowledge, skills, competencies, and attitudes of team members in concepts that are key to team success is essential. Exemplars presented here represent well-tested curricula from which organizations can benefit. Partners in academic and service settings can facilitate the development and implementation of evidence-based curricula as well as ongoing coaching, mentoring, and role modeling for successful teamwork to provide team-based care that will impact the health of patients, families, and communities. In the next chapter, we will discuss how to leverage the success of teams across organizations and communities.

QUESTIONS FOR THOUGHT

1. How do the team leadership training programs described in this chapter differ from those that your team has used for initial or continued development? Would a formal team leadership development program be of value to your team? How?
2. After analyzing skill gaps in your team, describe the components of the team training programs in this chapter that might be helpful to your team in filling those skill gaps.
3. How might your team use formal team leadership training programs to enhance their competencies in the areas of change management, conflict resolution, or developing strategy?

Leverage of Nursing and Health Care Team Results

TEN

Leveraging Productive Nursing and Health Care Teams Inside and Outside of the Organization

It's what you learn after you know it all that counts.
—*John Wooden*

LEARNING OBJECTIVES

1. Describe the process of self-advocacy for teams.
2. Identify the elements of successful communication of a team's strategic value with stakeholders.
3. Analyze how storytelling may enhance the communication of a team's strategic value.
4. Discuss how external funding opportunities may leverage the investment that organizations have made in team development.
5. Illustrate how return on investment (ROI) in teams can be demonstrated.

The term "leveraging" seems to appear everywhere in current-day leadership discussions. Organizations try to "leverage their resources." States try to "leverage their political power." Individuals try to "leverage their position for advancement." But what does leveraging really mean in the context of current health care organizations and teams? This chapter introduces the concept of "leverage" as it applies to teams, and describes a variety of methods for optimally using resources, which is what leveraging is all about. Demonstrating the strategic value of the team to the organization and to outside entities and finding opportunities for continued support of the team through team self-advocacy involve creating conversations about the team's work, and demonstrating the team's passion for what it does as a team. Attention to communication of the team's strategic worth both within and outside of the organization will guide team leaders to demonstrate the ROI in a high-performing team.

WHAT IS "LEVERAGING"?

The simplest definition of "leverage" or "leveraging" is using something to its best advantage. Although this simple definition might be helpful to some, within the context of teams and organizations, the definition presented by BusinessDictionary.com is more illustrative of the power of leveraging for teams and organizations. Their definition of leveraging, "the ability to influence a system, or an environment, in a way that multiplies the outcome of one's efforts without a corresponding increase in the consumption of resources"(www.businessdictionary.com/definition/leverage.html#ixzz2BSc2poNb), allows the team to see the real power of leveraging their work. After all, what organization would not want to increase the outcomes of the efforts to build and maintain high-performing teams without increasing their output of resources to do so? The team can leverage its work in a variety of ways. Self-advocacy, creating conversations about the team's work, and demonstrating team passion for its work are a great place to start.

SELF-ADVOCACY

In trying to leverage their work, teams need to advocate for themselves in a variety of situations. The term "self-advocacy" is a common term in the disability literature. Teams can learn much from the conceptualization of self-advocacy posited by the disability advocacy community. In her article *Self-Advocacy: Know Yourself, Know What You Need, Know How to Get It*, James (2012) defines self-advocacy as "the ability to understand and effectively communicate one's needs to other individuals. Learning to become an effective self-advocate … is all about educating the people around you" (p. 1). Although James is specifically addressing the disability advocacy community in this article, teams need to learn the same skills, to communicate their needs, skills, and unique contributions by educating others around them. Consider the following case in which a team educates its chief executive officer (CEO) of its unique contributions to the organization, and how those skills can be leveraged beyond the original intent of the team.

An interprofessional team of nurses, pharmacists, physicians, allied health professionals, and health sciences students and faculty have been working together for over a year to improve the process of medication reconciliation in a large hospital system. The problem of a lack of understanding of the treatment plan for medications was identified by the organization and the team in every unit of the organization. Not only were there gaps in understanding what medications a patient should be receiving within the organization, the processes for transfer of that understanding between referring organizations like skilled nursing homes, primary care centers, and specialty clinics were also fraught with chances for errors. The problem was resulting in increased medication errors in the organization, an alarming number of patients leaving the organization with prescriptions that were in conflict with the medications that they had at home, and increased call backs to the hospital by referring providers for clarification of medications postdischarge. The team worked together, along with a variety of partners and stakeholders from within and outside of the organization, to develop, negotiate, implement, and evaluate a streamlined process for medication reconciliation, enhanced by technology, which would follow the patient. The process was immensely successful, leading to a threefold decrease in medication errors in the organization as well as enhanced postdischarge outcomes.

During the adjourning phase of its work, the team members began a discussion of what they had learned during their work together. Although all had learned much about the medication reconciliation process, the team was proud of what it had learned about working together as a team, developing trusting alliances and partnerships with stakeholders, negotiating within and across systems for change, and evaluating their work. Backed by confidence in its abilities, the team began to think about how these skills might be applied in other areas of the organization. Several of the team members began a discussion of efforts at the organizational level to reduce 30-day readmissions to the organization. The problem was similar to that of medication reconciliation in that it was a complex systems issue, and spanned the boundaries of systems, as many readmissions were occurring from partner organizations like skilled nursing facilities, primary care centers, and specialty clinics. The team believed that they could leverage their knowledge and skills, developed during their previous work together, to address the readmission problem. The team developed a self-advocacy plan to optimize the use of their talents in the organization.

This example demonstrates how the skills of a team are translatable across problems faced by the organization. Self-advocacy plans can help others recognize those translatable skills.

To create a self-advocacy plan, teams will want to attend to *understanding their skills*, the *potential areas where these skills could be applied*, and *communicating these opportunities to key leaders in the organization*.

Understanding Skills

Chapter 3 addressed the importance of recognizing skills of team members that will enhance the work of the team during the formation of a team. Once the team has been working effectively together, team members have developed an entirely new set of skills that should be acknowledged and recognized. The team should spend time identifying those skills that have been enhanced and developed during their work together. A prime time for doing the work of skill identification is during team evaluation (as discussed in Chapter 7).

Identification of Other Areas Where Skills Could Be Applied

During the team evaluation process, teams should be intentionally asking the questions: How do these skills translate into other areas of our work? How could we use these skills in different ways to solve different problems? How can we share these skills with others in our organization? Is it possible for us to use the skills we have developed as a team to mentor other teams? To develop new teams? To stay together as a team and leverage our knowledge and skills in other areas of the organization?

Communicating Skills to Key Leaders

This step in the self-advocacy process is probably the most difficult for teams. After all, we have all been told not to "blow our own horns." However, this step, although the most difficult, is the most important step in the process of self-advocacy and leveraging the team's skills and talents. Without communication to key leaders of the team's unique skills, those skills will likely go unnoticed. In our case study of the medication reconciliation team, the team will be known as just that, the team that solved the medication reconciliation problem, unless they share the skills and talents that they have developed in the process as a team with others outside of the team.

Teams can approach the communication of their skills and talents with leaders of the organization in a variety of ways. Regardless of the form that communication takes, communication about the skills and talents of the team should be consistent, with all team members agreeing on the skill set that will be highlighted and presented. Communication plans for self-advocacy should be systematic, with the team agreeing upon who will communicate what to whom in the organization. It goes without saying that all team communications should be easy to understand, that anyone who hears about or reads about the skills and talents developed by the team will understand the communication. Use of flowery language and jargon should be avoided. The communication plan must fit the organization's culture and respect organizational lines of communication. For instance, it would not be appropriate for a team to ask to discuss their skills and talents with the chairperson of the Board of Directors for an organization if they have not already discussed this with the CEO. Finally, the communication plan for self-advocacy must be manageable for the team and also for those who will be the targets of communication. A too ambitious plan for communication may be detrimental to the team's success, especially if that plan calls for immense amounts of time spent by team members on creating multiple reports, presentations, and papers. Simple is best in this case. The team should develop a streamlined plan that will allow the members to best describe the skills that they have acquired, how those skills can be applied in other ways in the organization, and to the right people in the organization at the right time.

COMMUNICATION OF THE STRATEGIC VALUE OF TEAMS WITHIN ORGANIZATIONS

In Chapter 5, we discussed channels for communication about the team's work together both inside and outside of the organization. Although this discussion focused primarily on the work of the team, and not on "selling" the skills of the team to others, some of the same mechanisms for communication will work in the case of communicating for team self-advocacy purposes. Remember that the purpose of this communication is the demonstration of the strategic value of continued investment in or support of the team.

Specific methods of communication of strategic value to a team will depend upon the purpose and intended audience. For instance, a targeted article in a company newsletter or magazine, or a brief video segment shown on corporate-produced television or websites might work to get broad attention for the skills of the team, and may result in others recognizing the value of those skills in solving problems that the team has not yet identified. Email blasts may serve the same purpose. However, if the purpose of the team is to self-advocate for leveraging its skills with very specific application to a particular problem in the organization, the team will want to strategically target its communication plan to those who have authority over that problem. This group might include managers, directors, or chief executives. Direct methods of communication, in the form of brief personal e-mails, a short presentation at an executive level meeting, or a meeting one on one (or one on many) between the stakeholder and the team may be most appropriate. In this case, the same rules of communication apply—be consistent with the message, make your communication easy to understand, and provide manageable amounts of information. Lessons learned from the political advocacy community include:

1. *Make an appointment.* The stakeholders you are interested in engaging are busy people. They will be able to focus much more on the team's presentation if they have the time set aside to focus. Catching the director in a hallway between meetings will not be as effective as having even a short, uninterrupted block of time for the team to advocate for leveraging its skills in other places in the organization.
2. *Show up on time.* Be sure that all team members who will be present for the discussion with the stakeholder are able to attend the meeting on time and stay for the entire meeting. If some members are not available to do so, they should not plan to attend the meeting. Late arrivals and early departures are distracting and may give the impression that the team is not united in its cause.
3. *Be prepared to wait.* Again, stakeholders are busy people. They may run late. Do not let that discourage your team or affect the positivity with which the team approaches the stakeholder.

4. *Introduce your team and mention the general reason for the meeting.* Plan to provide a succinct and clear summary of the work that your team has done and why you are meeting today.
5. *Start on a positive note.* Promote the work that your team has done together and the skills that have been developed in a positive light. Clearly present how you as a team believe that the skills that you have developed are translatable to other issues within the organization. Show how continued support of the team can help the organization meet strategic goals of the organization. Very explicitly volunteer the services of the team to solve those problems that you have identified as amenable to your skills as a team.
6. *Listen and respond.* Be prepared to hear questions from the stakeholder. He or she will want to understand your skill set, and if you have presented in a compelling way, will be thinking through the steps in engaging your team to solve the problem you have identified.
7. *Stay on message.* Agree as a team that you will stay on message. Although it may be a rare occasion that team members get to interact with leaders high in the organization, this should not be a time when team members opt to begin a discussion of dissatisfaction with the newest salary guidelines.

Source: Adapted from the American Association of University Professors (2012).

FACTS TELL, STORIES SELL

When planning to communicate the strategic value of the team to organizational stakeholders, the old marketing adage "facts tell, stories sell" is true. Teams who use stories to sell their value can increase the impact that they have on stakeholders exponentially. Throughout this chapter, we have talked about the power of stories and storytelling for teams. In Chapter 6, we introduced the concept of using storytelling to engage team members and remember the purpose and impact of their work together. In that chapter, the idea of using stories to make connections among team members was presented. Teams can expand these techniques to make connections outside of the team, to have others connect to their work and their value.

Stories convey passion and allow people to make powerful connections between the story and their own lives, or the lives or circumstances of their organization. A good story taps into the emotions of the audience, connecting them in a strong way to the work of the team.

More important, a good story can help others see what the team has gone through since they have been together, how they have grown, matured, settled conflict, and succeeded. Stories can help the team share the good and bad they have learned—the lessons learned by the team can serve immense value for others. Teams can develop their own stories through following some simple guidelines.

1. *Engage your audience.* Make the story relevant to the purpose of your communication. The team who is self-advocating for continued support of the organization should tell a story that demonstrates clearly its strategic value to the organization.

2. *Always have a story ready for any circumstance.* All team members should be able to tell a story about the team's successes from their perspective. These stories should be able to be delivered in 1 minute, 5 minutes, 15 minutes, or longer depending on the circumstance and audience. Bottom line—have a story available that will allow each team member to convey his or her passion for the work of the team.

3. *Make sure your story has a hero.* All good stories have a hero. Think about every fairy tale or Hollywood movie you have ever seen. There is a hero. In your team's stories, the hero might be the team. But, the hero may also be a key stakeholder who made a difference in the work of the team, a team sponsor, or the patients and families who were impacted by the work of the team. Regardless of who the hero is, make sure you have clearly identified the conflict or dilemma faced by the hero, and how they overcame challenges to lead to a happy ending.

4. *Make sure that your story reflects your emotions and passions.* Do not be afraid to express the passion with which your team has undertaken its work or the strong emotions that have led you to this point. These are the types of stories that engage others, and allow them to relate and learn.

5. *If your team does not have good storytellers, invest in some education.* Although storytelling is powerful, it must be done well to be effective in your organization. If your team does not possess skills in storytelling, as with any other skill gap, the team has a choice. The team can develop that skill, or can go outside of the team to recruit members who have that skill. Because stories should be authentic to the team, the team will most likely choose to develop the skill within the team. Numerous web resources exist for storytelling; a quick Internet search will provide hundreds. A dynamic website with links to a variety of storytelling

resources has been developed by Dr. Elizabeth Figa (2012) at the University of North Texas and is available at www.courses.unt.edu/efiga/STORYTELLING/StorytellingWebsites.htm.

EXTERNAL OPPORTUNITIES TO LEVERAGE TEAM SUCCESS

When a team has been successful in an organization, one of the imperatives of the team should be to share that knowledge outside of the organization. A variety of mechanisms exist for sharing the team's success outside of the organization. For instance, depending on the team's purpose for existing, the team may want to present the *products* of their work together at professional meetings. They may want to publish their work in a professional journal. These scholarly forms of communication allow the dissemination of the *products* of the team's work with an audience that may be able to learn from the team's success and replicate the results in other organizations. Plenty of resources are available to those teams that may want to develop an abstract and paper detailing its *products* for peer review for presentation and/or publication. In this chapter though, we are focusing on how to leverage the *skills* of the team in innovative ways. So, the focus here will be on how we can share the *skills* of the team outside of the organization.

One of the most common ways to share the skills of the team is through *consultation* with other teams. Teams that have developed successful processes for teamwork are in high demand in most organizations. Through self-advocacy in professional networks, teams can begin to "get the word out" that they are available for consultation to teams in other organizations—not to solve organizational problems, but rather to help teams develop in effective ways.

Many organizations have professional education or corporate development departments as part of their organization. Teams that wish to share their expertise in team development, facilitation, and effectiveness may propose that they develop a continuing-education program or series of programs for interested teams. This approach could actually be entrepreneurial for teams and allow them to bring in funds to the organization to support continued team development.

Teams may also offer their services to local colleges and universities, teaching students how to develop, support, and guide effective teams. Because teamwork is an important competency at all levels of nursing and health professional education, this may be an opportunity for teams to not only provide a real-life perspective about team development, but may also be an opportunity to influence the next generation of health care providers in their development of teamwork competencies.

Finally, teams may want to explore the development of more in-depth team development curricula to be offered for aspiring teams. As organizations realize the power of successful teams in facilitating the accomplishment of their goals, team training programs are in high demand. Teams can take what they have learned and help other developing teams systematically advance the skills that they have developed during their work together. Some sample curricula for team development training programs are found in the Appendix of this book. Teams can modify these to reflect their own experiences and the needs of developing teams.

FUNDING OPPORTUNITIES AS LEVERAGE MECHANISMS

In some cases, the continuation or expansion of the work of teams is predicated upon continued financial support of the work of the team. Many times, teams have developed products on a small scale that could be leveraged and tested in larger populations or organizations for effectiveness. Funders external to the organization may be interested in providing that continued support. For instance, a recent call for applications from the National Institutes of Health sought proposals to "develop infrastructure that will leverage existing health care delivery systems to efficiently test the effectiveness of treatment, preventive and services interventions to improve care for people with mental disorders ... propose a research infrastructure that demonstrates the ability to identify, recruit and enroll large patient populations into effectiveness trials, harmonize electronic medical record data across multiple integrated systems for research use, pool data for common analyses, and build capacity for the collection and storage of biologic material" (NIH, 2010, p. 1). An established team that had been working together within a complex health care delivery system on improvement of care and services for those with mental health disorders would be well suited to apply for these funds, allowing them to leverage their work on an even larger scale, while creating new infrastructure to support future study of care interventions. As an aside, the funding available for one site for this particular call for applications was $9 million over 3 years! Another example of the use of external funding sources to leverage the work of teams comes from the FCC (Federal Communications Commission). In 2007, the FCC created a Rural Healthcare Pilot Program designed to provide support for technology infrastructure to meet the needs of rural health care providers. The greatest value of the pilot program was the ability of health care providers who had previously been working on the issue of technology access in small teams or on their own to work together to create statewide and regional networks. An interesting finding from the program was that grantees learned that the process of establishing networks was difficult, so most participants did not spend the bulk of their funding to construct new networks of their own, rather where there were already existing services, they leveraged those services by entering into agreements with existing providers to connect health care facilities in a region or state. Where services were not available, they used the power of their partnerships to convince service providers to build facilities and develop pricing strategies that increased access to rural care providers (FCC, 2007). This is an excellent example of how funding can expand the work of a team into a broader partnership while maintaining the original goal of creating an information technology infrastructure for rural health care.

How can teams use these funding sources to their best advantage to leverage their work? The process of grantsmanship is complex, but can essentially be summarized in several steps. These include:

- Identification of grant opportunities
- Matching grant purposes to the team's mission
- Crafting the application for funding
- Receipt of funding
- Stewardship of funding support

Identification of grant opportunities: The sources of potential funding for teams to leverage their work are many. The challenge for teams is identification of those sources of funding. Primary sources of funding that teams may want to access include private donors, foundations, industry, and/or government. Many health care organizations, hospitals, and colleges/universities have a development department, and may have their own foundation. This would be the optimal starting point for identification of potential donors who may have an interest in the work of the team. A recent team that worked on the development of an introduction to the career of nursing web program was funded by a private donor who had an interest in supporting middle and high school students who were interested in health careers; the donor also had an ongoing relationship with the university. A meeting with the donor and the team was set up by the development officer at the university and the team presented their project. After some discussion, the donor decided that the passion shown by the team and the way that their project matched his interests made the project worthy of investment. The donor provided a $30,000 check to the organization to support the team's work. In the absence of a Development department in the team's organization, the team can work with the organizational leadership to recognize and approach potential donors. Grateful patients, community members, and local businesses may be sources of these donations.

Identification of foundations that could potentially fund the work of the team is a matter of searching the community, state, and national grant databases. For instance, the organization *Grantmakers in Health* represents membership of over 240 foundations that provide grants and funding for health-related issues. By visiting their website www .gih.org/index.cfm, a team can access the websites of each of those funders, read about their funding priorities, and find open application opportunities. Online foundation directories are available, for instance, the *Foundation Directory Online* (www.fconline.foundationcenter.org) created by the Foundation Center, is a subscription service that may also be available at public libraries. Teams can search these databases by state, community, or topical area to find foundations whose missions match the mission of the team.

Industry funders are typically identified by teams from professional relationships that may have been developed with product vendors or pharmaceutical representatives, for example. If a team has, for example, developed a project that uses a product in an innovative way to solve a system's problem, the team may want to approach the product vendor about the potential of leveraging their work through their industry's support. Product vendors may not have grant funding that they personally control; however, they may be able to direct the team to the industry representative who could guide them through the grant process.

Finally, government funders are a source of small and large funding that teams may want to consider in order to leverage their work on a larger scale. State funding may be available from a variety of sources, including the legislature, the governor's office, or from specific agencies. Teams can visit their state websites to find out information specific to initiatives in their state. The federal government has developed a central storehouse for information on over 1,000 grant programs and all discretionary grants offered by the 26 federal grant-making agencies in the federal government. This database is found at www07.grants .gov/index.jsp, and provides access to approximately $500 billion in annual awards. Teams can search this database by topical area, by granting agency, or by the grant number if available to the team. Teams can sign up for alerts from this database by visiting the subscription page at www07.grants.gov/applicants/email_subscription.jsp. Teams can choose to receive an RSS (rich site summary) feed of new grant opportunities and grant news, or receive daily e-mail alerts for new grant opportunities, or to receive alerts when grant opportunities are released in their topic of interest (USDHHS, 2012).

Matching grant purposes to team's mission: The team will want to assure that the purpose of the grant, typically found on the grantor's webpage or other printed materials, matches closely with the team's mission. Typically, it is a waste of time to seek grant funding from an agency in which the link between their purpose for awarding the grant funds is not aligned with the work that the team will try to accomplish. For instance, if a grant's goal is to support changes to prevent or reduce exposure to harmful environmental toxins and improve the health of a community, it would likely not be appropriate to submit an application for the further development and expansion of a project to support breastfeeding in a hospital setting. Although breastfeeding may improve the health of a community, the call for applications is specific, and there should be a clear link between the application of the team and the purpose of the grant.

Crafting the application for funding: There are hundreds of guides available in print and on the Internet to teach teams to learn how to write a successful grant application. A web resource that team's may want to access, as it is a compendium of grants-writing resources, is available from the USDA (U.S. Department of Agriculture) and is found at www.nal.usda.gov/ric/ricpubs/fundguide.html. This database houses up-to-date information on funding processes, grant databases, grant-writing resources on the web and in publication, funding newsletters, and topic-specific information especially about health-related funding. Any of these resources would be valuable to a team as it creates an application for funding.

Receiving the funding and stewardship: If an application for funding is approved, the team will expect to receive funding from the grantor. The grantor may want to negotiate a change to the proposed budget; if so, the team should enter into those negotiations with an understanding that it should not negotiate a reduction of funding if the reduction will not allow them to develop the product that they have proposed in their application. As a grantee, the team also has the responsibility of being a good steward of the funds. This means that teams must only use the funds for which they were intended in the way that was described in the grant application. The team must provide the services or programs they proposed unless they receive explicit permission from the granting agency to do otherwise. The team must collect data needed for reports to the grantor, and must provide those reports as requested and on time. Finally, if funds are not expended for the project, the team must assure that the funds are returned to the funder in a timely way. Good stewardship of funding will allow the team to be in a good position to apply for future funds to leverage its work.

ROI for Teams

ROI is a financial term that denotes the evaluation of the benefit of a program over and above the costs of that program. For teams, an ROI analysis can help the team to document its value to an organization through justification of the costs spent on the team's development and support. ROI is typically calculated as a percentage, and any percentage greater than 0 denotes that the investment has returned more to the organization than it cost. The simple formula for ROI is:

$$\text{Simple ROI} = \frac{\text{Gains or Benefits} - \text{Investment or Program Costs}}{\text{Program Costs}} \times 100$$

The advantages of calculating an ROI for teams are many. These include credibility with organizational leadership, documentation of strategic advantages realized through team support, and team motivation. Showing that the investment in a team has value beyond the initial investment is powerful. The major disadvantage of using ROI in health care is that some program benefits may be intangible and difficult to translate into cost. For example, it may be difficult, but not impossible, to place a monetary value on leadership training for a team. However, if skills in negotiation, collaboration, and conflict management developed during leadership training avert the loss of a surgical practice that threatens to move to a competitor organization, the benefit is able to be expressed in terms of real dollars—which would be equal to the value of the surgical cases to the organization in a year. The investments or costs in this instance would be the cost of the leadership training, among others.

To calculate ROI, a team will need to be able to identify the gains or benefits as a result of its work, as well as the costs of or investments to its work. The simplest way to demonstrate this is through the following case:

> A team of public health experts work together to develop a county immunization plan after an outbreak of meningitis. The plan is implemented, and the team undertakes an ROI analysis. For program benefits, the team analyzes the number of hospitalizations for meningitis in the 6 months prior to the implementation of the immunization plan and the number of hospitalizations during the 6 months after immunizations. They estimate the average length of stay for those hospitalizations and the average cost of a hospitalization for meningitis. These analyses serve as the program benefits—the decrease in number of hospital days and subsequent decreased costs for care. They also calculate the investments or program costs. These include the cost of staff for planning and implementation (number of staff × number of hours × salary per hour), overhead costs for provision of services, supply and immunization costs, and training costs. Once they have captured all program costs, they calculate the ROI using the formula provided previously. The simple ROI for this program is 83%.

Teams can use more complex ROI formulas as well, and there are a number of worksheets, spreadsheets, and examples of the use of ROI in health care and professional development available in published texts as well as on the Internet. Jack Phillips, PhD, is considered to be a leading expert in ROI analysis, and his ROI Institute is a valued source of information, tools, case studies, publications, and education programs regarding the use of ROI in a variety of sectors (www.roiinstitute.net/). Of particular interest in health care may be the tool available on this site called ROI Analysis Plan, found under the Healthcare Tools section. The direct link to this tool is www.media.roiinstitute.net/tools/2007/05/24/ROIAnalysisPlan.pdf.

SUMMARY AND NEXT STEPS

Demonstrating the strategic value of the team to the organization and to outside entities and finding opportunities for continued support of the team through team self-advocacy involves creating excitement about the team's work in a variety of ways and demonstrating the team's passion for what it does as a team. Leveraging the work that the team has done can provide added value to its organization as well as to other organizations. The ability to disseminate and expand the team's work through attainment of continued funding and operational support can expand the value of the team even further. Attention to communication of the team's strategic worth both within and outside of the organization will guide team leaders to demonstrate the ROI in a high-performing team. In the next and final chapter of the book, we will apply and expand the concepts of teamwork to their broadest application: coalitions, alliances, and partnerships.

QUESTIONS FOR THOUGHT

1. Think about the skills developed in a current team. How could these specific skills be applied to other complex problems within your organization?
2. Develop a plan for self-advocacy of a team. How will you demonstrate the team's strategic value to the organization? How can you communicate how the organization can leverage the investment that they have made in the team in the future?
3. Tell the compelling story of the impact that your team has had on a specific problem in the organization. Highlight the teaming skills that have been developed during your work together and how these might serve the organization well in the future.
4. Identify three sources of potential funding for your team's continued work. Consider how you might craft a proposal to at least one of these funding sources in the next 3 months to support your work.
5. Identify the elements that would be necessary to evaluate your organization's ROI in your team. What elements will you need to consider? Is there existing data that will help you to analyze ROI? If not, how can you plan to collect these data?

ELEVEN

Nursing and Health Care Partnership Building for Sustained Team Results

Let's make a dent in the universe.
—Steve Jobs

LEARNING OBJECTIVES

1. Describe how the concept of partnership is related to the concept of teamwork.
2. Analyze the similarities between partnerships and teams, especially in the areas of mission, vision, ground rules, goals, objectives, evaluation, and adjournment.
3. Identify how partnerships can be built from team successes.
4. Describe methods to sustain partnerships.

Early in Chapter 1, the concept of partnership was introduced as closely related to the concepts of teams and teamwork. Definitions of partnerships lead us to conclude that similar to teaming, partnerships imply shared responsibilities and accountability. Although teams are typically considered to be intraorganizational, partnerships are usually considered to be interorganizational. In fact, Roberts (2004) defines a partnership as occurring when "two or more organizations come together for mutual benefit" (p. 1). The World Health Organization defines a partnership as "a collaborative relationship between two or more parties based on trust, equality and mutual understanding for the achievement of a specified goal. Partnerships involve risks as well as benefits, making shared accountability critical" (WHO, 2009, p. 1).

Just like teams, successful partnerships require specific skills and strategies. The common traits found in partnerships include:

- Collaboration
- Trust
- Equality
- Mutual understanding
- A stated goal
- Shared accountability

These common traits sound very similar to those we have discussed for teams throughout this text. Successful teams and partnerships collaborate in a trusting way to meet their common goals while treating each other as equals. Mutual understanding of the goals, rules, and expected outcomes are reached through communication, negotiation, and action. Although teams are accountable to other team members and the organization, partners are accountable to the partnership, but also possess a sense of accountability back to the original organization. Not unlike teams, Suchman, Walker, and Botelho (1998) believe that there are three constants in partnerships. These include:

> *Relationships*: Partnerships are about developing, maintaining, and sustaining relationships. For the partnership to be successful, relationships must be forged, maintained, and sustained.
>
> *Understanding*: Suchman and colleagues (1998) believe that "one must strive to understand the perspectives of others to be an effective partner" (p. 2). That shared understanding allows partners to leverage the strength of the partnership to its fullest extent.
>
> *Shared decision making*: For a partnership to thrive, all partners must be involved in decisions that impact the partnership. During decision making, partners will necessarily not only be thinking about the partnership but will also be considering the impact of decisions on their own organization as well. Although this perspective and dual allegiance makes shared decision making more complicated, it also strengthens the partnership through enhancing commitment to decisions of the group.

Given their similarities, we can apply much of what we have focused upon in this text related to teams to the concept of partnerships. In fact, creating, nurturing, and supporting partnerships take many of the same skills as those of creating, nurturing, and supporting teams. In this chapter, we will apply what we now know about teams to partnerships—from establishing purpose to creation of successful partnerships. We will also look at the benefits offered and challenges posed when working in partnerships. Finally, we will examine unique models of partnership, including virtual partnerships and emerging models of partnership, for instance, the Accountable Care Organization (ACO) model.

PURPOSE OF PARTNERSHIPS

Teams are formed to meet a purpose. Likewise, partnerships are developed from a common need, to use the power of the partners to meet a common goal. Typically, partnerships grow from an identified need, an intractable problem that cannot be solved by a single person or organization. The problems are such that one organization cannot possibly address the problem alone. For example, an organization may note that there is inequity in the way providers are being reimbursed in their organization under a new state Medicaid managed care policy. Nurse practitioners are not recognized as independent practitioners as required by state law. Although this single organization may want to "take on" the state Medicaid program, the organization may also opt for developing a partnership with other affected organizations to add strength to its position. Another example of a partnership with a clear purpose is the Partnership for Patients: Better Care, Lower Costs initiative, launched by the Obama Administration. This public–private partnership is designed to improve the quality, safety, and affordability of health care for all Americans. The Partnership for Patients brings together leaders of major hospitals, employers, physicians, nurses, and patient advocates along with state and federal governments in a shared effort to make hospital care safer, more reliable, and less costly.

This partnership has two goals:

- *Keep patients from getting injured or sicker.* By the end of 2013, preventable hospital-acquired conditions would decrease by 40% compared to 2010. Achieving this goal would mean approximately 1.8 million fewer injuries to patients with more than 60,000 lives saved over 3 years.
- *Help patients heal without complication.* By the end of 2013, preventable complications during a transition from one care setting to another would be decreased so that all hospital readmissions would be reduced by 20% compared to 2010. Achieving this goal

would mean more than 1.6 million patients would recover from illness without suffering a preventable complication requiring rehospitalization within 30 days of discharge (Healthcare.gov, 2012a, 2012b).

Achieving these goals will save lives and prevent injuries to millions of Americans and has the potential to reduce health care costs tremendously. Goals like these are perfectly suited to partnerships—these problems cannot be addressed by a single organization, but rather, partnerships must include stakeholders at every point along the continuum of education, care, and payment.

BENEFITS AND RISKS OF PARTNERSHIPS

The organization or organizations that enter into partnerships believe that perceived benefits of acting together as partners outweigh the risks of joining together. Key to the success of partnerships is a perceived benefit by the partners. Those benefits might include parameters such as sharing resources, saving time, learning from one another, expanding creativity, or increased legitimacy. These benefits must outweigh the risks to partnership, which might include loss of power, reputation, or resources.

BARRIERS TO EFFECTIVE PARTNERSHIPS

Although there are obvious benefits to effective partnerships, there are also many barriers. These barriers will be familiar to readers of this text, as many of the same barriers will hinder the success of a team. Barriers to successful partnerships include:

- Lack of clear purpose of the partnership or lack of buy-in or understanding of purpose
- Lack of understanding of partner roles
- Lack of support from partner organizations
- Differences of philosophies or conflict in acceptable ways of working
- Lack of commitment
- Unequal and/or unacceptable balance of power and control
- Key interests or stakeholders who are missing from the partnership
- Hidden agendas
- Lack of clear and consistent communication
- Lack of a method to evaluate or monitor the work of the partnership

■ Failure to learn from successes or failures
■ Conflict of commitments

Source: Adapted from Compassion Capital National Resource Center (2010).

STEPS TO CREATING SUCCESSFUL PARTNERSHIPS

Similar to the development of teams, the development of partnerships must be intentional. Therefore, several steps should be considered when creating a partnership. These include:

1. **Emphasize the importance of leadership**
   One of the first steps that a partnership will want to undertake will be the selection of a leader. Partners need to understand that leadership is not just centered in the person who has been selected, but also in his or her organization. Partners must be comfortable with their choice and trust that the leader and the organization will act in the best interest of the partnership. Conversely, the organization of the selected leader must be comfortable with and empowered by his or her own organization to serve as the leader for the partnership.

2. **Be clear about partner roles and responsibilities**
   Partners must recognize that each organization will have varied degree of involvement at different times in the partnership, based on skills, resources, and organizational demands. Partners should develop clarity from the outside about partnership expectations, roles, and responsibilities. Partners should be sure that the right stakeholders are involved in the partnership. Partners should also analyze skill gaps and identify how they will fill those gaps for the partnership's success.

3. **Recognize and embrace differences in organizational culture among partners**
   All partners will come to the partnership bearing their own unique organizational culture, rules, and behaviors. The partnership must recognize this diversity and embrace it. Failure to do so will lead to conflict among the partners.

4. **Ensure clarity of purpose**
   Just as in teams, leaders should ensure the partnership is built on a shared vision and mutually agreeable goals. All partners should understand the purpose of the partnership and be a part of developing goals that will help them meet the intended outcomes of

the partnership. Even more important than in teams, in a partnership, shared commitment is essential to future success. Once goals and objectives are developed, they should be communicated widely, within the partnership organizations, and, if appropriate, outside of those organizations. Although the partnership can acknowledge that each partner has her or his own organizational strategic goals, the goals of the partnership are equally as important to all members.

5. **Ensure a level of commitment from each partner organization**
Each organization in the partnership needs to have the commitment of leaders in their organization to the goals of the partnership, and the continued pursuit of those goals. Support may be in the form of explicit acknowledgment of partnership goals, or through human or financial resources committed to the goals. Recognizing the strengths of each partner in the organization will be helpful in gaining support. For instance, if one partner organization has great strength in public relations, and another in networking, the partnership should use those partner's strengths to meet the partnership goals, and should ask for commitment from those partners to use those strengths. Partners can learn from teams—capitalize on strengths and fill skill gaps for maximum success.

6. **Develop and maintain trust**
As in teams, trust is an imperative to success in a partnership. Actions to develop trust in partners are similar to those in teams—professional behavior, communication using a variety of mediums, transparency, giving feedback, handling conflicts, and the development and adherence to ground rules will help partners to develop and maintain trust throughout their relationship.

7. **Develop an evaluation plan**
As in teams, evaluation of the partnership will be key to maintaining motivation, continued development, and leveraging the partnership. All partners should agree early in their work together how they are to measure their success and how they will use these measurements to continually improve their partnership.

8. **Recognize the opportunity to leverage what the partnership has learned**
In Chapter 10, we discussed how teams might leverage their work together and share what they have learned beyond the organization. Partnerships should be prepared to do similar work—sharing their successes but also what they have learned from and about

working together. Developing and maintaining a partnership is hard work. Partners should celebrate their successes, and share their experiences widely, so that others might benefit from what they have learned from working together.

UNIQUE PARTNERSHIP MODELS

Similar to teams, partnerships can be operationalized in many ways. Some of the emerging, unique models of partnership are using technology to virtually drive their work together and expand their reach. Others have emerged with health care reform as methods not only to improve care quality but also to increase access, decrease costs, and impact the safety of the care environment. Examples of how partnerships have thrived when supported in the virtual environment as well as in an era of health care reform are included here.

Virtual Partnerships

Just because potential partners are not in close geographic proximity to one another does not mean that a powerful partnership cannot exist. If the preexisting need for a partnership exists, that is, there is an intractable problem that one organization alone cannot fix, distance should not prohibit partnership. Likewise, if the intractable problem is complex or crosses nontraditional boundaries, partnership should not be ruled out, but rather, technology can be embraced to facilitate partnership. The steps previously described still apply—partnerships must have a leader, a clear purpose, shared trust, a commitment to action, and a way to evaluate and leverage their results—albeit those steps might be accomplished in a different way than at face-to-face meetings. Consider the following example of a virtual partnership:

> The director of a health care workforce research center at a large university became increasingly aware in his work that there was a need for reliable workforce information related to the nursing workforce for decision making at the state and national level. This need went beyond what his workforce center could provide as a state-supported entity primarily engaged in looking at workforce issues in his own state. Through his network of other leaders in the health care workforce, he knew that there was an incredible amount of

work that was ongoing and completed regarding the nursing workforce, but the efforts to find all of these data were sometimes monumental—they were housed in universities, professional organizations, regulatory boards, workforce centers, state and health departments, labor departments, and other government entities. Some were published in journals, in conference proceedings, in reports to the legislature, or in other media. Having the ability to reliably access these data would assist researchers in comparing their work to that of others, would assist policymakers to evaluate the impact of potential legislation on the nursing workforce, would help workforce planners learn from the past and forecast into the future, and would allow those in workforce development to respond to evidence related to trends in the nursing workforce in the development of on-the-ground initiatives. Tackling the issue of getting all of the data in one place for easy access was more than one workforce center could handle. Therefore, the development of a nursing workforce clearinghouse was born.

The concept was discussed at major meetings of nursing workforce leaders, and buy-in to the purpose was obtained. Partners were sought from across the United States, including workforce centers, nursing leaders in education, practice, and research, large professional organizations, and state and national regulators. Because of widespread geographic diversity of these leaders and their organizations, a virtual partnership was born. The partners followed the steps of partnership development contained in this chapter, including establishing a leader and lead organization; refining their purpose; defining goals, strategies, and deliverables; establishing trust and regular communication; and developing an evaluation plan for their success. Through this successful virtual partnership, a virtual clearinghouse for nursing workforce data was developed and made operational. The partnership eventually was leveraged into a professional organization of nursing workforce centers that now maintains the clearinghouse that avails members of the ability to post reports and other materials, provides links to all nursing workforce centers, and allows members to query other members about pressing nursing workforce issues in their states.

This case is a prime example of the power of a strong partnership. Partners followed best practices in partnership development, used the strengths of the partners to accomplish their goals, and later leveraged that success into a different kind of lasting partnership.

Another example of a partnership that made use of virtual tools, not only for collaboration within the partnership but also to expand partnerships between clinicians and patients, is the New Health Partnership, managed by the Institute for Health Care Improvement (IHI, n.d.). This Robert Wood Johnson Foundation (RWJF)-funded initiative encompassed multilevel components directed by experts from leading organizations in chronic care and patient-centered care research with the specific goal to "inspire profound change in health care for all."

The mission of New Health Partnerships was to support and manage an online community of partners by providing information, resources, opportunities for discussion, and real-world examples. The goals were to:

- Support a patient- and family-centered approach to health care in which patients with chronic conditions, families, and providers work together
- Offer resources and tools to clinicians, patients, family members, and communities so that they could effectively collaborate in self-management support
- Build community-wide support for collaborative self-management
- Use up-to-date technologies to assist providers, patients, family members, and communities in improving chronic care
- Provide clinicians and administrative leaders with tools and examples to evaluate the business case for collaborative self-management support
- Encourage the active participation of all in New Health Partnerships (IHI, n.d.)

The partners in the project designed, tested, refined, and spread best practices in self-management support. The website for the New Health Partnerships contains patient and family as well as health care provider toolkits for self-management, plus stories of success from the partners. Organizational partners were diverse, but each brought to the table an interest in improving the care of patients with chronic disease. Distances between partners were bridged through the use of virtual technologies.

Policy-Driven Partnerships

When the Patient Protection and Affordable Care Act was passed by the U.S. Congress and signed into law by President Barack Obama on March 23, 2010, numerous opportunities for partnerships were created. The most prominent of all of these opportunities is found in the accountable care organization (ACO) provisions of the law. On March 31, 2011, the Department of Health and Human Services (DHHS) released new rules to help doctors, hospitals, and other providers better coordinate care for Medicare patients through ACOs. ACOs create incentives for health care providers to work together to treat an individual patient across care settings—including doctor's offices, hospitals, and long-term care facilities. The Medicare Shared Savings Program will reward ACOs that lower growth in health care costs while meeting performance standards on quality of care and putting patients first. Although a complete discussion of ACOs is outside of the scope of this chapter, it is important to note that policy development for ACO expansion has included the key provisions of partnerships. The policy provides for improving coordination and communication among physicians and other providers and suppliers through ACOs, which will help improve the care Medicare beneficiaries receive, while also helping lower costs. According to the analysis of the proposed regulation for ACOs, Medicare could potentially save as much as $960 million over 3 years.

ACOs as Partnerships

Under the proposed rule, an ACO refers to a group of providers and suppliers of services (e.g., hospitals, physicians, and others involved in patient care) that will work together to coordinate care for the patients they serve. The goal of an ACO is to deliver seamless, high-quality care for Medicare beneficiaries. The law requires each ACO to include health care providers, suppliers, and Medicare beneficiaries on its governing board. Under this model of partnership, ACO partners share the risk and benefits of provision of coordinated care. Under the proposed rule, Medicare would continue to pay individual health care providers and suppliers for specific items and services as it currently does. The Centers for Medicare and Medicaid Services (CMS) would also develop a benchmark for each ACO against which ACO performance is measured to assess whether it qualifies to receive shared savings or to be held accountable for losses. The amount of shared savings depends on whether an ACO meets or exceeds quality performance standards. The proposed rule links the amount of shared savings an ACO may receive to its performance on quality standards. The rule proposes quality measures in five key areas that affect patient care:

- Patient/caregiver experience of care
- Care coordination
- Patient safety
- Preventive health
- At-risk population/frail elderly health

The proposed rule sets out performance standards for each of these measures and a proposed scoring method, including proposals to prevent providers in ACOs from being penalized for treating patients with more complex conditions (Healthcare.gov, 2012a, 2012b).

ACOs then are a good example, if implemented correctly, of a partnership model. Groups of organizations come together to solve the problem of providing high-quality care to Medicare beneficiaries. The partnership will require planning, collaboration, communication, and trust to succeed. Shared risks and rewards provide motivation for all partners. Relationships, communication, and shared decision making, all hallmarks of a successful partnership, will be required to achieve the outcome of improved patient care quality at a lesser cost.

SUMMARY AND NEXT STEPS

Partnerships and teams possess many similar characteristics. Leaders can translate knowledge of how to intentionally develop, support, and sustain effective teams to develop, support, and sustain effective partnerships. Partnerships are somewhat more complicated than typical teams in that partners have a shared alliance with the partnership but also with their own organization. Although this shared alliance may create challenges and barriers to partnerships, with purposeful application of team competencies to partnerships, leaders can facilitate partnership success.

The next step for readers of this book is to use the knowledge gained in practice. When faced with a challenge that requires the work of a team or partnership, be intentional about the selection of team members, how skills are used and enhanced, and how teamwork is implemented within the unique environment of the organization. Take time to plan to evaluate your work together, not only the product of your work but also the processes that were necessary to accomplish your goals. And finally, consider how you can leverage your work in the world around you—by sharing your knowledge with others or expanding the scope and direction of your team or partnership. The end result of intentionally creating and leading teams in health care will be improved care for our patients, families, and communities.

QUESTIONS FOR THOUGHT

1. Think about a partnership that you have been involved with in your work or your community. What was the purpose of the partnership? How were relationships built and capitalized upon in the partnership? How was trust built? What were the strategies that the partners used for shared decision making?
2. You have just been selected as the leader for your partnership. What will your first steps be in the partnership? In your organization?
3. Consider opportunities that surround you in your work and community to develop partnership relationships. What do those opportunities have in common? How might you capitalize on emerging technologies, reimbursement strategies, or models of care to develop partnerships in those areas?
4. As you think about teams and partnerships, what do you think are the main differences in challenges to maintaining and sustaining each? The similarities?

APPENDIX

Web Resources

Resources noted in this book are available for use by organizations, leaders, and teams in their work. Some of these resources are available for purchase; others are available for download or access free of charge. This appendix is designed to provide links to essential resources, arranged by their appearance in the chapters in the book. Every attempt has been made to ensure the integrity of the web addresses included here. All are current at the time of publication.

In addition to these resources, readers may find additional team resources by searching the Internet or at their local library. A number of applications for smartphones related to team development, team management, and team evaluation are also available by searching "app stores." Finally, teams may find other valuable advice about teams through a number of business and health care blogs, interest groups, and professional societies available on the web.

CHAPTER 1: THE INTERSECTION OF TEAMS, PARTNERSHIPS, AND LEADERSHIP IN NURSING AND HEALTH CARE

- Institute of Medicine (IOM) report on *The Future of Nursing: Leading Change, Advancing Health.* Available at www.iom.edu/ Reports/2010/The-Future-of-Nursing-Leading-Change-Advancing-Health.aspx
- National League for Nursing Education Competencies Model. Available at www.nln.org/facultyprograms/competencies/pdf/ comp_model_final.pdf
- American Association of Colleges of Nursing Essentials Series. Available at www.aacn.nche.edu/education-resources/essential-series
- Quality and Safety Education for Nurses. Available at www.qsen .org

- Core Competencies for Interprofessional Practice Expert Panel Report. Available at www.aacn.nche.edu/education-resources/ipecreport.pdf

CHAPTER 2: ELEMENTS OF EFFECTIVE NURSING AND HEALTH CARE TEAMS AND PARTNERSHIPS

- Myers–Briggs-Type Inventory (MBTI), Consulting Psychologists Press. Available at www.cpp.com
- Team Management Systems Team Management Profile Questionnaire. Available at www.tms.com.au

CHAPTER 3: GETTING STARTED: BUILDING A STRONG TEAM

- The MindTools Organization. Available at www.mindtools.com
- Team Management Systems Linking Skills. Available at www/tms .com.au/linkingskills.html

CHAPTER 4: TEAM STRATEGIES FOR SUCCESS IN NURSING AND HEALTH CARE ENVIRONMENTS

- Microsoft SharePoint. Available at www.sharepoint.microsoft.com/ en-us/Pages/default.aspx
- DropBox™. Available at www.dropbox.com/teams
- Team Charter. Available at www.acquisition.gov

CHAPTER 5: WORKING AS A TEAM WITHIN THE NURSING AND HEALTH CARE ORGANIZATION

- Organizational Culture Assessment Instrument (OCAI). Available at www.ocai-online.com
- Organizational Profile Model. Available at www.timothy-judge .com/OCP.htm
- Scott and colleagues (2003) article reviewing Organizational Culture assessment instruments. Available at www.ncbi.nlm.nih.gov/pmc/ articles/PMC1360923/#b24

CHAPTER 6: PLANNING FOR NURSING AND HEALTH CARE TEAM AND PARTNERSHIP SUCCESS

- Icebreakers from Team Building USA. Available at www .teambuildingusa.com/business-meeting-icebreakers

- Daily Scrum Guidelines. Available at www.scrum.org
- Stay on track with scrum meetings. Available at www .effectivemeetings.com/teams/teamwork/scrum.asp
- Coverdale Organization Systematic Approach. Available at www .coverdale.co.uk
- Facilitate Pro™. Available at www.facilitate.com
- MeetingSense®. Available at www.meetingsense.com
- Online training resources for root-cause analysis. Available at www.healthinsight.org/Internal/Incident_Investigation-RCA .html
- The W.K. Kellogg Foundation Logic Model. Available at www .wkkf.org/knowledge-center/resources/2006/02/WK-Kellogg-Foundation-Logic-Model-Development-Guide.aspx

CHAPTER 7: MEASURING TEAM AND PARTNERSHIP SUCCESS IN NURSING AND HEALTH CARE ENVIRONMENTS

- Comprehensive Assessment of Team Member Effectiveness. Available at www.catme.org.
- Team Evaluation Survey template. Available at www.123contactform .com/free-form-templates/Team-Evaluation-37436

CHAPTER 8: PERIODIC MAINTENANCE FOR THRIVING NURSING AND HEALTH CARE TEAMS AND PARTNERSHIPS

- The Traffic Light Team Coaching Model. Available at www .coachingconnect.co.uk
- IDEO. Available at www.ideo.com
- CMS Innovation Center. Available at www.innovations.cms.gov/ initiatives/Innovation-Advisors-Program/index.html
- The World Café. Available at www.theworldcafe.com
- SCAMPER: Improving Products and Services. Available at www .mindtools.com/pages/article/newCT_02.htm

CHAPTER 9: TEAM LEADERSHIP TRAINING AND DEVELOPMENT PROGRAM EXEMPLARS

- West Virginia Nursing Leadership Institute. Available at www .wvnli.org
- Agency for Health Care Quality and Research TeamSTEPPS model. Available at www.teamstepps.ahrq.gov/about-2cl_3.htm

- Geriatric Interdisciplinary Team Training. Available at www .gittprogram.org

CHAPTER 10: LEVERAGING PRODUCTIVE NURSING AND HEALTH CARE TEAMS INSIDE AND OUTSIDE OF THE ORGANIZATION

- Storytelling resources. Available at www.courses.unt.edu/efiga/ Storytelling/StorytellingWebsites.htm
- Grantmakers in Health. Available at www.gih.org/index.cfm
- Foundation Directory Online, Foundation Center. Available at www.fconline.foundationcenter.org
- Federal grant opportunities. Available at www07.grants.gov/index .jsp
- Federal grant opportunities e-mail alert sign up. Available at www07.grants.gov/applicants/email_subscription.jsp
- USDA grant writing resource compendium. Available at www.nal .usda.gov/ric/ricpubs/fundguide.html
- Return on Investment Institute. Available at www.roiinstitute.net

CHAPTER 11: NURSING AND HEALTH CARE PARTNERSHIP BUILDING FOR SUSTAINED TEAM RESULTS

- Partnerships for Patients. Available at www.healthcare.gov/ compare/partnership-for-patients
- Institute for Health Care Improvement (IHI): New Health Partnerships. Available at www.ihi.org/offerings/Initiatives/PastStrategic Initiatives/NewHealthPartnerships/Pages/default.aspx

References

Agency for Healthcare Research and Quality (AHRQ). (n.d.-a). *Patient safety primer: Root cause analysis.* Retrieved from http://psnet.ahrq.gov/primer.aspx?primerID=10

Agency for Healthcare Research and Quality. (AHRQ). (n.d.-b). *TeamSTEPPS program.* Retrieved from http://www.teamstepps.ahrq.gov/about-2cl_3.htm

Aiken, L. H., Clarke, S. P., & Sloane, D. M. (2002). Hospital staffing, organization, and quality of care: Cross-national findings. *Nursing Outlook, 50*(5), 187–194.

Aiken, L. H., Clarke, S. P., Sloane, D. M., Sochalski, J., & Silber, J. H. (2002). Hospital nurse staffing and patient mortality, nurse burnout, and job dissatisfaction. *Journal of the American Medical Association, 288*(16), 1987–1993.

Aiken, L. H., Smith, H. L., & Lake, E. T. (1994). Lower Medicare mortality among a set of hospitals known for good nursing care. *Medical Care, 32*(8), 771–787.

Aiken, L. H., Sochalski, J., & Lake, E. T. (1997). Studying outcomes of organizational change in health services. *Medical Care, 35*(11 Suppl.), 6–18.

Amabile, T. (1998, September–October). How to kill creativity. *Harvard Business Review,* pp. 77–87.

American Association of Colleges of Nursing. (2006). *The essentials of doctoral education for advanced nursing practice.* Retrieved from http://www.aacn.nche.edu/education-resources/essential-series

American Association of Colleges of Nursing. (2008). *The essentials of baccalaureate education for professional nursing practice.* Retrieved from http://www.aacn.nche.edu/education-resources/essential-series

American Association of Colleges of Nursing. (2011). *The essentials of master's education in nursing.* Retrieved from http://www.aacn.nche.edu/education-resources/essential-series

American Association of University Professors. (2012). *How to visit a congressional office.* Retrieved from: http://www.aaup.org/AAUP/GR/lobbytools/How+to+Visit+a+Congressional+Office.htm

Anderson, N., & West, M. (1998). Measuring climate for work group innovation: Development and validation of the team climate inventory. *Journal of Organizational Behavior, 19*(3), 235–258.

Association of American Medical Colleges. (2011). *Core competencies for interprofessional collaborative practice: Report of an expert panel.* Washington, DC: Interprofessional Education Collaborative.

Bacon, C. T., Hughes, L. C., & Mark, B. A. (2009). Organizational influences on patient perceptions of symptom management. *Research in Nursing and Health, 32,* 321–334.

Bae, S., Mark, B., & Fried, B. (2010). Impact of nursing unit turnover on patient outcomes in hospitals. *Journal of Nursing Scholarship, 42*(1), 40–49.

Bag, P., & Pepito, N. (2012). Peer transparency in teams: Does it help or hinder incentives? *International Economic Review, 53*(4), 1257–1286.

Baker, D., Day, R., & Salas, E. (2006). Teamwork as an essential component of high reliability organizations. *Health Services Research, 41*(4 part 2), 1576–1598.

Baker, D. P., Gustafson, S., Beaubien, J., Salas, E., & Barach, P. (2005, April). *Medical teamwork and patient safety: The evidence-based relation. Literature review.* AHRQ Publication No. 05-0053. Rockville, MD: Agency for Healthcare Research and Quality. Retrieved from http://www.ahrq.gov/qual/medteam

Baldwin, D. (1996). Some historical notes on interdisciplinary and interprofessional education and practice in the USA. *Journal of Interprofessional Care, 10,* 173–187.

Bantel, K. A., & Jackson, S. E. (1989). Top management and innovations in banking: Does the composition of the top team make a difference? *Strategic Management Journal, 10,* 107–124.

Barker, W., Williams, T., Zimmer, J., VanBuren, C., Vincent, S., & Pickrel, S. (1985). Geriatric consultation teams in acute hospitals: Impact on back-up of elderly patients. *Journal of the American Geriatrics Society, 33*(6), 422–428.

Battles, J. B., Kaplan, H. S., Van der Schaaf, T. W., & Shea, C. E. (1998). The attributes of medical event-reporting systems: Experience with a prototype medical event-reporting systems for transfusion medicine. *Archives of Pathology & Laboratory Medicine, 122*(3), 231–238.

Bergman, P. (2009, April 28). How to counter resistance to change. *Harvard Business Review Blogs.* Retrieved from http://blogs.hbr.org/bregman/2009/04/how-to-counter-resistance-to-c.html

Cable, D. M., & Judge, T. A. (1997). Interviewers' perceptions of person-organization fit and organizational selection decisions. *Journal of Applied Psychology, 82,* 546–581.

Caldwell, D., Chatman, J., O'Reilly, C., Ormiston, M., & Lapiz, M. (2008). Implementing strategic change in a health care system: Importance of leadership and change readiness. *Healthcare Management Review, 33*(2), 124–133.

Cameron, K., & Quinn, J. (2011). *Diagnosing and changing organizational culture.* San Francisco: Jossey-Bass.

Campbell, D., & Hallam, D. (1994). *Campbell–Hallam team development survey.* Arlington, VA: Vangent, Inc.

Cannon-Bowers, J., & Salas, E. (2000). *Making decisions under stress: Implications for individual and team training.* American Psychological Association. Retrieved from http://www.ahrq.gov/qual/medteam/medteamfig1.htm#a

Carrasco, V. (2009). *Building collaborative capacity across institutional fields: A theoretical dissertation based on a meta-analysis of existing empirical research.* Retrieved from http://www.scribd.com/viviancarrasco/d/16969792-Building-Collaborative-Capacity

Center for Creative Leadership. (2007). *CCL White Paper: The state of teams.* Retrieved from http://www.ccl.org/leadership/pdf/research/StateOfTeams.pdf

Cho, T. S., & Hambrick, D. C. (2006). Attention patterns as mediators between top management team characteristics and strategic change: The case of airline deregulation. *Organization Science, 17*(4), 453–469.

Clark, G. (2002). Organisational culture and safety: An interdependent relationship. *Australian Health Review, 25*(6), 181–189.

Clarke, S., Sloane, D., & Aiken, L. (2002). Effects of hospital staffing and organizational climate on needlestick injuries to nurses. *Journal of Public Health, 92*(7), 1115.

Collins, J., & Porras, J. (1996, September–October). Building your company's vision. *Harvard Business Review.*

Compassion Capital National Resource Center. (2010). *Partnerships: Frameworks for working together*. Washington, DC: National Resource Center for U.S. Department of Health and Human Services.

Contratti, F., Ng, G., & Deeb, J. (2012). Interdisciplinary team training: Five lessons learned. *American Journal of Nursing, 112*(6), 47–52.

Cowan, M. J., Shapiro, M., Hays, R., Afifi, A., Vazirani, S., & Ward, C. et al. (2006). The effect of a multidisciplinary hospitalist physician and advanced practice nurse collaboration on hospital costs. *Journal of Nursing Administration, 36*(2), 79–85.

Cox, I. W., Plagens, G. K., & Sylla, K. (2010). The leadership–followership dynamic: Making the choice to follow. *International Journal of Interdisciplinary Social Sciences, 5*(8), 37–51.

Cronenwett, L., Sherwood, G., Barnsteiner, J., Disch, J., Johnson, J., Mitchell, P., …, Warren, J. (2007). Quality and safety education for nurses. *Nursing Outlook, 55*(3), 122–131.

Cronenwett, L., Sherwood, G., Pohl, J., Barnsteiner, J., Moore, S., Sullivan, D., …, Warren, J. (2009). Quality and safety education for advanced nursing practice. *Nursing Outlook, 57*(6), 338–348.

Dahl, C. (2000, November 30). Natural leader. *Fast Company*.

Downey, M. (2003). *Effective coaching*. Cheshire, UK: Texere Publishing.

Drucker, P. (2007). *The effective executive*. New York: Butterworth-Heinneman.

Edgar, L. (1999). Nurses' motivation and its relationship to the characteristics of nursing care delivery systems: A test of the Job Characteristics Model. *Canadian Journal of Nursing Leadership, 12*(1), 14–22.

Eickenberry, K. (2007). *Elements of high performing teams. The sideroad*. Retrieved from http://www.sideroad.com/Team_Building/high-performance-teams.html

Elenkov, D. S., Judge, W. Q., Jr., & Wright, P. (2005). Strategic leadership and executive innovation influence: An international multi-cluster comparative study. *Strategic Management Journal, 26*(7), 665–682.

Erickson, T. (2009). *Do you have the collaborative capacity you need?* Retrieved from http://www.wikinomics.com/blog/index.php/2009/06/28/do-you-have-the-collaborative-capacity-you-need

Esposito-Herr, M., Persinger, K., Regier, A., & Hunt, S. (2009). Partnering for better performance: The nursing–finance alliance. *American Nurse Today, 4*(4).

Ettner, S., Kotlerman, J., Abdemomnem, A., Vazirani, S., Hays, R., & Shapiro, M. et al. (2006). An alternative approach to reducing the costs of patient care? A controlled trial of the multi-disciplinary doctor–nurse practitioner (MDNP) model. *Medical Decision Making, 26*, 9–17.

Falk, A., & Ichino, A. (2006). Clean evidence on peer effects. *Journal of Labor Economics, 24*, 38–57.

Federal Communications Division. (2007). *Rural healthcare pilot program*. Retrieved from http://www.fcc.gov/guides/rural-health-care-pilot-program

Figa, E. (2012). *Storytelling websites and resources*. Retrieved from http://www.courses.unt.edu/efiga/Storytelling/StorytellingWebsites.htm

Finkelstein, S., & Hambrick, D. (1990). Top management team tenure and organizational outcomes. *Administrative Science Quarterly, 35*, 484–503.

Firth-Cozens, J. (2001). Cultures for improving patient safety through learning: The role of teamwork. *Quality Health Care, 10*(Suppl. 2), 26–31.

Flynn, L., Liang, Y., Dickson, G., Xie, M., & Suh, D. (2012). Nurses' practice environments, error interception practices and inpatient medication errors. *Journal of Nursing Scholarship, 44*(2), 180–186.

Foundation Center. (n.d.). *Foundation directory online.* Retrieved from http://fconline.foundationcenter.org

Frankel, A., Gardner, R., Maynard, L., & Kelly, A. (2007). Using the communication and teamwork skills (CATS) assessment to measure health care team performance. *Joint Commission Journal on Quality and Patient Safety, 33*(9), 549–558.

Fulmer, T., Flaherty, E., & Hyer, K. (2003). The geriatric interdisciplinary team training program. *Gerontology and Geriatric Education, 24*(2), 3–12.

Gage, M. (1998). From independence to interdependence: Creating synergistic healthcare teams. *Journal of Nursing Administration, 28*(4), 17–26.

Generic team charter template. (n.d.). Retrieved from http://www.acquisition.gov

Geriatric Interdisciplinary Team Training. (n.d.). Retrieved from http://gittprogram.org

Gillies, R. R., Shortell, S. M., Casalino, L., Robinson, J. C., & Rundall, T. G. (2003). How different is California? A comparison of U.S. physician organizations. *Health Affairs*, doi: 10.1377/hlthaff.w3.492

Gittell, J. H. (2002). Coordinating mechanisms in care provider groups: relational coordination as a mediator and input uncertainty as a moderator of performance effects. *Management Science, 48*(11), 1408–1426.

Gittell, J., Fairfield, K., Bierbaum, B., Head, W., Jackson, R., Kelly, ..., Zuckerman, J. (2000). Impact of relational coordination on quality of care, postoperative pain and functioning and length of stay: A nine hospital study of surgical patients. *Medical Care, 38*(8), 807–819.

Gittell, J., Godfrey, M., & Thistlewaite, J. (2012, October). Interprofessional collaborative practice and relational coordination: Improving healthcare through relationships. *Journal of Interprofessional Care* (epub ahead of print).

Glenaffric Ltd. (2007). *Six steps to effective evaluation: A handbook for programme and project managers.* Retrieved from http://www.jisc.ac.uk/media/documents/funding/project_management/evaluationhandbook0207.pdf

Global diversity and inclusion: Fostering innovation through a diverse workforce. (2011). Forbes Insights. Retrieved from http://www.forbes.com/forbesinsights/innovation_diversity/index.html

Griffin, R., & Moorhead, G. (2011). *Organizational behavior.* Boston: South-Western College Publishers.

Hackman, J., & Oldham, G. (1976). Motivating through the design of work: Test of a theory. *Organizational Behavior and Human Performance, 16*, 250–279.

Hatch, M., & Schultz, M. (1997). Relations between organizational culture, identity and image. *European Journal of Marketing, 31*(5/6), 356–365.

Havens, D., Vasey, J., Gittell, J., & Lin, W. (2010). Relational coordination among nurses and other providers: Impact on the quality of patient care. *Journal of Nursing Management, 18*, 926–937.

Healthcare.gov. (2012a). *Accountable care organizations: Improving care coordination for people with Medicare.* Retrieved from http://www.healthcare.gov/news/factsheets/2011/03/accountablecare03312011a.html

Healthcare.gov. (2012b). *Partnerships for patients.* Retrieved from http://www.healthcare.gov/compare/partnership-for-patients

Heskett, J. (2011). Manage the Culture Cycle. World Financial Review, (Sept–Oct), 2–7.

Hirsh, S., & Kummerow, J. (1998). *Introduction to type in organizations* (3rd ed.). Palo Alto, CA: Consulting Psychologists Press.

Hoegl, M., & Parboteeah, K. P. (2006). Autonomy and teamwork in innovative projects. *Human Resource Management*, 45(1), 67–79.

Inculcating culture. (2006). *Economist, 378*(8461), Retrieved from http://www.economist.com/node/5380462

Institute for Health Care Improvement (IHI). (n.d.). *New health partnerships.* Retrieved from http://www.ihi.org/offerings/Initiatives/PastStrategicInitiatives/NewHealthPartnerships/Pages/default.aspx

Institute of Medicine. (1999). *To err is human: Building a safer health system.* Washington, DC: National Academies Press.

Institute of Medicine. (2010). *The future of nursing: Leading change, advancing health.* Washington, DC: Institute of Medicine.

Interprofessional Collaborative Expert Panel. (2011). *Competencies for interprofessional collaborative practice: Report of an expert panel.* Washington, DC: Interprofessional Education Collaborative.

James, N. (2012). *Self-advocacy: Know yourself, know what you need, know how to get it.* Retrieved from http://www.wrightslaw.com/info/sec504.selfadvo.nancy.james.htm

Johanson, G., Eklund, K., & Gosman-Hedstrom, G. (2010). Multidisciplinary team-working with elderly persons living in a community setting: A systematic literature review. *Scandinavian Journal of Occupational Therapy*, 17(2), 101–116.

Kalisch, B. J., Curley, M., & Stefanov, S. (2007). An intervention to enhance nursing staff teamwork and engagement. *JONA: Journal of Nursing Administration*, 37(2), 77–84.

Katzenbach, J. R., & Smith, D. K. (1993). *The wisdom of teams: Creating the high performance organization.* Boston, MA: Harvard Business School Press.

Kotter, J., & Heskett, J. (2011). *Corporate culture and performance.* New York: Free Press.

Lambrou, P., Kontodimopoulos, N., & Niakas, D. (2010). Motivation and job satisfaction among medical and nursing staff in a Cyprus public general hospital. *Human Resources for Health*, 8(26), 1–9.

Langhorne, P., Williams, B., Gilchrist, W., & Howie, K. (1993). Do stroke units save lives? *Lancet, 343*(8868), 395–398.

Larrabee, J., Withrow, M., Janney, M., Hobbs, G., Ostrow, C. L., & Durant, C. (2003). Predicting registered nurse job satisfaction and intent to leave. *Journal of Nursing Administration*, 33(5), 271–283.

Lemieux-Charles, L., & McGuire, W. L. (2006). What do we know about health care team effectiveness: A review of the literature. *Medical Care Research Review, 63*(3), 263–300.

Lewis, G., & Drife, J. (2004). *Why mothers die 2000–2002.* London: Royal College of Obstetricians and Gynecologists Press.

Mainstay Partners. (2011). *Leading enterprises turn to SharePoint to build productive social networks.* Retrieved from http://sharepoint.microsoft.com/en-us/resources/Pages/Whitepapers.aspx?Title=Leading+Enterprises+Turn+to+SharePoint+to+Build+Productive+Social+Networks&ResourceType=White+Paper

Marion, A. (Ed.). (2001). Organizational structure. In *Encyclopedia of Business and Finance* (Vol. 2). Farmington Hills, MI: Gale Cengage Learning. Retrieved from http://www.enotes.com/organizational-structure-reference

Mathis, K. (2011). *Setting measurable project objectives*. Retrieved from http://www. projectsmart.co.uk/pdf/setting-measurable-project-objectives.pdf

Mawji, Z., Stillman, P., Laskowski, R., Lawrence, S., Karoly, E., Capuano, T., & Sussman, E. (2002). First do no harm: Integrating patient safety and quality improvement. *Joint Commission Journal of Quality Improvement, 28*(7), 373–386.

Mazzocco, K., Petitti, D. B., Fong, K. T., Bonacum, D., Brookey, J., Graham, S., Lasky, R. E., …, Thomas, E. J. (2009). Surgical team behaviors and patient outcomes. *American Journal of Surgery, 197*(5), 678–685.

McCann, D. J. (2003). *The workplace behavior pyramid*. TMS Australia. Access e-book at http://www.tms.com.au/shop/ebk3.html

McCann, D. J. (2009). *The dynamics of high performing teams*. TMS Australia. Retrieved from http://www.tmsoz.com/files/PDF/Whitepapers/Dynamics-of-High-Performing-Teams-TMSOz.pdf

Meterko, M., Mohr, D., & Young, G. (2004). Teamwork culture and patient satisfaction in hospitals. *Medical Care, 42*(5), 492–549.

Mickan, S. M. (2005). Characteristics of effective teams: A literature review. *Australian Health Review, 29*(2), 211–217.

Mikes, J. (2010). *Team charters: What are they and what is their purpose. Life Cycle Engineering*. Retrieved from http://www.lce.com/Team_Charters_What_are_they_and_whats_their_purpose_360-item.html

MindTools. (2012). *SCAMPER: Improving products and services*. Retrieved from http://www.mindtools.com/pages/article/newCT_02.htm

MindTools. (n.d.). *Effective recruitment: Finding the best people for your team*. Retrieved from http://www.mindtools.com/pages/article/effective-recruitment.htm

Montes, F., Moreno, A., & Morales, V. (2005). Influence of support leadership and teamwork cohesion on organizational learning, innovation and performance: An empirical examination. *Technovation, 25*(10), 1159–1172.

Morey, J., Simon, R., Jay, G., & Rice, M. (2003). A transition from aviation crew resource management to hospital emergency departments: The Medteams story. In R. S. Jensen, (Ed.), *Proceedings of the 12th International Symposium on Aviation Psychology*, pp. 826–832.

Morgan, G. (2006). *Images of organizations*. Thousand Oaks: Sage.

Myers, I. B. (1998). *Introduction to type* (6th ed.). Palo Alto, CA: Consulting Psychologists Press.

Myers, I., McCaulley, M., Quenk, N., & Hammer, A. (1998). *MBTI manual (a guide to the development and use of the Myers–Briggs-type indicator)* (3rd ed.). Palo Alto, CA: Consulting Psychologists Press.

National Institutes of Health. (2010). *Leveraging existing health care networks to transform effectiveness research (U19)*. Retrieved from http://grants.nih.gov/grants/guide/rfa-files/RFA-MH-10-030.html

National League for Nursing. (2010). *NLN Education Competencies Model*. Retrieved from http://www.nln.org/facultyprograms/competencies/pdf/comp_model_final.pdf

O'Reilly, C., Chatman, J., & Caldwell, D. (1991). People and organizational culture: A profile comparison approach to assessing person-organization fit. *Academy of Management Journal, 34*(3), 487–516.

Offermann, L., & Spiros, L. (2001). The science and practice of team development: Improving the link. *Academy of Management Journal, 44*(2), 376–392.

Ohland, M. (2012). *Comprehensive assessment of team member effectiveness*. Retrieved from www.catme.org

Persily, C. (2010). *West Virginia Nursing Leadership Institute Team Development Program: Final report to the Robert Wood Johnson Foundation/Northwest Health Foundation Partners Investing in Nursing's Future Program*. Unpublished, available upon request.

Phillips, J. (n.d). *Return on investment institute*. Retrieved from http://www.roiinstitute.net

Pink, D. (2009). *Drive: The surprising truth about what motivates us*. New York, NY: Riverhead Books. Epub 2010 Oct 13.

Quality and Safety Education for Nurses. (2012). Retrieved from www.qsen.org

Quinn, R., & Rohrbaugh, J. (1981). A competing values approach to organizational effectiveness. *Public Productivity Review, 5*, 122–140.

Rafferty, A., Ball, J., & Aiken, L. (2001). Are teamwork and professional autonomy compatible, and do they result in improved hospital care? *Quality in Health Care, 10*(Suppl. II), ii32–ii37.

Rath, T. (2007). *StrengthsFinder 2.0*. New York, NY: Gallup Press.

Rath, T., & Conchie, B. (2009). *Strengths based leadership*. New York, NY: Gallup Press.

Robbins, S., & Judge, T. (2012). *Organizational behavior*. Saddle River, NJ: Prentice-Hall.

Roberts, J. (2004). *Alliances, coalitions and partnerships*. Canada: New Society Publishers.

Schein, E. (1990). Organizational culture. *American Psychologist, 45*(2), 109–119.

Schmidt, I., Claesson, C., Westerholm, B., Nilsson, L., & Svarstad, B. (1998). The impact of regular multidisciplinary team intervention on psychotropic prescribing in Swedish nursing homes. *Journal of the American Geriatrics Society, 46*(1), 77–82.

Scott, L. (2012). *Team coaching and feedback*. Retrieved from http://www.coaching-connect.co.uk

Scott, T., Mannion, R., Davies, H., & Marshall, M. (2003a). Implementing culture change in health care: Theory and practice. *International Journal for Quality in Health Care, 15*(2), 111–118.

Scott, T., Mannion, R., Davies, H., & Martin, M. (2003b). The quantitative measurement of organizational culture in health care: A review of the available instruments. *Health Services Research, 38*(3), 923–945.

Senge, P. (2006). *The fifth discipline: The art and practice of the learning organization*. New York, NY: Crown Business.

Shwaber, K., & Sutherland, J. (2011). *The scrum guide*. Retrieved from http://www.scrum.org/Portals/0/Documents/Scurm%20Guides/Scrum_Guide.pdf

Silverman, R. (2012, February 12). No more angling for the best seat; more meetings are stand-up jobs. *The Wall Street Journal*.

Singh, M. (n.d.). *Getting and estimating resource requirements*. Retrieved from http://www.projectminds.com/Article15.html

Slaikeu, K. (1996). *When push comes to shove: A practical guide to mediating disputes*. San Francisco: Jossey-Bass.

Smith, W. K., & Tushman, M. L. (2005). Managing strategic contradictions: A top management model for managing innovation streams. *Organization Science, 16*(5), 522–536.

Stay on track with scrum meetings. Retrieved from www.effectivemeetings.com/teams/teamwork/scrum.asp

Suchman, A., Walker, P., & Botelho, R. (1998). *Partnerships in healthcare: Transforming relational process.* Rochester, NY: University of Rochester Press.

Swyers, M. (2012). 7 reasons good teams become dysfunctional. *Inc.* Retrieved from http://www.inc.com/matthew-swyers/7-reasons-good-teams-become-dysfunctional.html

Takeuchi, H., & Nonaka, I. (1986, January–February). New product development game. *Harvard Business Review.*

Teasley, S., Covi, L., Krishnan, M., & Olsonino, J. (2002). Rapid software development through team co-location. *IEEE Transactions on Software Engineering, 28,* 671–683.

Thompson, L. (2003). Improving the creativity of organizational work groups. *Academy of Management Executive, 17*(1), 98–109.

Thorson, R. (2005). *Myers Briggs type awareness: Team building and personnel relations in the work place.* UMI Proquest. Retrieved from http://gradworks.umi.com/cgi-bin/redirect?url=http://gateway.proquest.com/openurl%3furl_ver=Z39.88-2004%26res_dat=xri:pqdiss%26rft_val_fmt=info:ofi/fmt:kev:mtx:dissertation%26rft_dat=xri:pqdiss:MR05105

3M Company. (1998). *Anatomy of great meetings.* Retrieved from http://www.3rd-force.org/meetingnetwork/files/meetingguide_anatomy.pdf

TMS Global. (n.d.). *The concepts: Linking skills.* Retrieved from http://www.tms.com.au/linkingskills.html

Toode, K., Routasalo, P., & Suominen, T. (2011). Work motivation of nurses: A literature review. *International Journal of Nursing Studies, 48*(2), 246–257.

Tuckman, B. W. (1965). Developmental sequence in small groups. *Psychological Bulletin, 63*(6), 384–399.

Tzeng, H., Ketefian, S., & Redman, R. (2002). Relationship of nurses' assessment of organizational culture, job satisfaction, and patient satisfaction with nursing care. *International Journal of Nursing Studies, 39*(1), 79–84.

USDA. (2012). *A guide to funding resources.* USDA, Rural Information Center National Agricultural Library. Retrieved from http://www.nal.usda.gov/ric/ricpubs/fund-guide.html

U.S. Department of Health and Human Services. (2012). Grants.gov. Retrieved from http://www.grants.gov

W.K. Kellogg Foundation. (2004). *Logic model development guide.* Battle Creek, MI: Author.

West, M. A. (1990). The social psychology of innovation in groups. In M. A. West & J. L. Farr (Eds.), *Innovation and creativity at work: Psychological and organizational strategies* (pp. 4–36). Chichester, UK: Wiley & Sons.

White, R. (1987). Managing innovation. *ELT Journal, 41*(3), 211–218.

WHO/African Partnerships for Patient Safety. (2009). *Building a working definition of partnership.* Retrieved from http://www.who.int/patientsafety/implementation/apps/resources/defining_partnerships-apps.pdf

Wiersema, M. F., & Bantel, K. A. (1992). Top management team demography and corporate strategic change. *Academy of Management Journal, 35,* 91–121.

Williams, M., Williams, T., Zimmer, J., Hall, W., & Podgorski, C. (1987). How does the team approach to outpatient geriatric evaluation compare to traditional care: A report of a randomized clinical trial. *Journal of the American Geriatrics Society, 35*(12), 1071–1078.

The world café presents café to go. (2008). Retrieved from http://www.theworldcafe.com

World Health Organization. (2009). *Building a working definition of partnership*. Retrieved from http://www.who.int/patientsafety/implementation/apps/definition/en

Xyrichis, A., & Ream, E. (2008). Teamwork: A concept analysis. *Journal of Advanced Nursing, 61*(2), 232–241.

Yun, S., Cox, J., Sims, H., & Salam, H. (2007). Leadership and teamwork: The effects of leadership and job satisfaction on team citizenship. *International Journal of Leadership Studies, 2*(3), 171–193.

Zimmer, J., Groth-Jincker, A., & McCusker, J. (1985). A randomized controlled study of a home health care team. *American Journal of Public Health, 75*(2), 134–141.

Zwarenstein, M., Goldman, J., & Reeves, S. (2009). Inter-professional collaboration: Effects of practice-based interventions on professional practice and healthcare outcomes. *Cochrane Database Systematic Review, 3*, CD000072.

Index

47472657R00153

Made in the USA
San Bernardino, CA
31 March 2017